I Never Held You

A book about miscarriage, healing, and recovery

Ellen M. DuBois

With Commentaries by Linda R. Backman, Ed.D., Licensed Psychologist and Grief Counselor, and a special chapter entitled *What is Reiki?* by Anna Pizzoferrato, certified Reiki and Shamballa Master/Teacher

Book Companion Website
http://www.miscarriagehelp.com

Contents

Parting Thoughts

Resources

Acknowledgments and a Note from Ellen

A special thank you to Dr. Linda Backman, who believed in me and this book enough to pour her heart and soul into it, often during a very busy schedule. My heartfelt thanks to Anna Pizzoferrato, who not only shares her expertise as a Reiki Master (in Part Two), but her painful recollection of living through not one, but *five* miscarriages. To Marnie Pehrson, published author and owner of SheLovesGod.com, for opening her heart and sharing her story and faith. To Mary Foster, my wonderful friend and confidant, whose story of miscarriage shows the devastating impact a complete lack of support after miscarriage causes. Having all suffered at least one miscarriage, we connected in a way that only women who have endured such a loss, ever could. A special thank you to my publisher, Sidney, who not only believed in this book when she published it as a small ebook over five years ago, but carried her belief in *I Never Held You's* message of hope and healing, catapulting it into the book you're reading now. She understood my vision of helping women worldwide who have suffered the pain and isolation of miscarriage, and has been the springboard to the next level.

I began this book as a way of reaching out to those who miscarried and didn't know where to turn or what to do with their feelings. Why? Because I was at a total loss when I miscarried and couldn't find anything that spoke directly to me and my loss. I needed something to make me say, "I feel exactly the same way. Finally, someone understands and can help. I am not alone." I wanted to provide, through this book, a means of connection between us. I believe that through connection comes the beginning of healing. Isolation only serves to make a person feel worse and less understood.

My journey first led me to Dr. Linda Backman. She is a licensed psychologist and specializes in grief counseling. What began as a collaborative writing project, soon turned into a deeper healing experience for myself. Through Linda's words and expertise, she showed me that life is a continual process of change, growth, and acceptance of yourself—no matter what point you're at in your life. I cannot thank Linda enough, and I know her words will leave an indelible mark within you.

As one who doesn't believe in coincidence, I know my journey 'led' me to Anna and Marnie, too. Their stories, combined with what went on to be lives that would heal and help many, needed to be told. In finding them, I discovered something about myself, perhaps all of us. Quite often, living through pain prepares us for something better down the road, although we can't see it during our experience. I didn't. I'd be willing to say the other women mentioned didn't. I've learned that within all of us lies an amazing ability to get through the adversities in life, and an ever-growing capacity to experience the joys as we heal and continue on our individual paths—wherever they may lead us.

I speak to you as a woman who has lived what you have lived. I want you to feel like you're listening to a friend who not only knows of, but feels the pain and confusion in your heart and mind, and doesn't dismiss it.

Dr. Backman speaks to you not only as a professional, offering sound words of encouragement and advice, but also as woman who has lived what you have lived.

It is my sincerest hope that you, the woman who has miscarried, will somehow be led to this book. My wish is for the words on these pages to reach into your heart and soul, making you feel far less alone and far more understood.

Most importantly, my greatest desire is of *hope and healing* for you. There *is* life after miscarriage—a *quality* life—and Dr. Backman and I want to hold your hand and help lead you down the road to recovery.

There is no greater step than that of the first.

The best to you on your journey,
Ellen

Forward

Dr. Linda Backman

I am a doctor, a psychologist doctor, and I do know what it is to have a baby born at 26 weeks of pregnancy, live a very short length of time, and die. This is what some call a Newborn Death. The pain and grief that go hand in hand following such a loss are familiar to me. On that very day some thirty years ago, when our second child was born and died, life took a rather different route. And I know, beyond the shadow of a doubt, it was meant to change. Did I recognize the change as I struggled with all of the whys and wherefores? Of course not, the destination and the course were absolutely clouded by pain and confusion.

I never held you, second son of mine, but what is clear is that you came, you left, and life was shoved in an entirely new direction.

Approximately, six weeks following Adam's birth and death, emotional hills and valleys had become the norm for me. In fact, my distress had become pronounced enough that my husband and I felt a call to the obstetrician was in order. Neither my doctor, nor the psychiatrist, nor my friends understood grief involving the loss of a baby and could explain what was happening to me. I honestly thought I was "losing it." Often I have described the state I was in as feeling like the "emotional flu." Another apt description would be I felt as though someone had taken a wool blanket, soaked it in water, and laid it on top of me. The weight I felt was indescribable.

The next question might be: How did I grow beyond the mire which held me down? And a further question would be: What led me to become a psychologist, presently having been in practice for nearly twenty-five years? At this juncture, without being boastful, I have established a public agency devoted to the grief surrounding child death, served on hospice boards, led grief support groups, presented at national and international conferences on grief, and provided many other means of support to grieving individuals. What I want to share here is what I felt step by step, how I managed to transform pain into love and life change, and where the journey can lead.

So, please stay with Ellen and me as we walk you through our grief and beyond. In addition, you will come to understand what others experience and what is painful, but normal along the road of grieving for yourself, your family and your child. I invite you to read all of what we offer in one sitting or simply "bite, chew, and swallow" one page at a time. I can't tell you how long your acute pain will last...perhaps six months...perhaps eighteen months or more...but what I can confidently say is if you truly allow yourself to recognize your feelings and label them as grief over the loss of your child, you will gradually follow the journey to a place of understanding and evolution.

Come with us to a newfound level of knowing life.

Part One

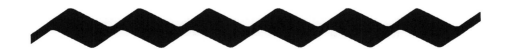

Miscarriage

I'm not a doctor, but I know what it is to miscarry. I'm not a psychiatrist, but I can tell you about the pain and grief that accompany a miscarriage. I'm not an expert in anything except this: I've had a miscarriage, and I know firsthand what it feels like. I know the pain and guilt. I've lived those days when you wonder why and come up empty-handed. I know how lonely and isolated you can feel. I know what it's like to have your grief dismissed—because there was never a baby 'seen.' And, I have learned that there's a lot of grieving, growing, letting go, and moving forward that needs to happen.

For your sake.

I also know that when I tried to find any books or material that dealt with the emotional roller coaster ride after a miscarriage, I couldn't find anything other than a pamphlet at a doctor's office or an article in a magazine. I felt worse when in bookstores because all of the books in the Parenting or Child sections were about having a baby—*not* losing one. It only served to magnify my pain.

It's taken me fifteen years to be able to write this—fifteen years of peaks and valleys, highs and lows, grieving and questioning, blaming and crying. I write not to take away your pain but to validate it and help diminish it. I write in the hope of reaching those of you who, like me, miscarried and don't know where to turn. To those of you out there desperately searching for someone to say, "You're not alone in this and your feelings are very real," I write these words. I have lived it.

Notice I didn't say *forgetting*. If anyone says to you, "It's time to forget this," I can say that I've never *forgotten* my miscarriage, and you don't need to, either. I've moved past it, but not without a lot of crying, self-blame, questioning myself and my faith, and feeling an overall sense of 'what could have been.'

If I were in the middle of my grief, anger, and despair, I could not write these words. My head wasn't clear enough after my miscarriage and for some time after that. I was too absorbed in my loss to know how to articulate my feelings—and, most importantly, I hadn't taken the journey towards recovery. Without that journey, which only time can offer, I would not have the ability to support you in your time of need.

My Story

When I was four and a half months pregnant, I was filled with feelings of excitement, joy, fear, and wonder. I had been married about a year and a half, and although it was an unplanned pregnancy, an immediate bond formed between my unborn and I. There were days when I would rest my hand on my slightly swollen stomach and smile, thinking of the life inside me. No, we didn't plan this baby, but I was going to give it all the love in the world and then some.

Nothing else mattered. I knew we'd manage.

One day, while my husband, (at the time), was away on business, I noticed a small amount of blood on some toilet paper. Instinct kicked in and said, "This isn't right. Call your doctor." There was no pain, no large amounts of blood—but the feeling that something was wrong was unshakable.

My sister and I ended up at the hospital where they performed an ultrasound. I stared at the monitor while the doctor pointed at an image that I could barely see through my tears. His words will forever ring in my ears: "The fetus is no longer viable." *Viable?* What did that mean? I could tell by the look on the doctor's face that it wasn't good.

"What does viable mean?" I asked. My heart raced as I awaited what I knew was the answer, but prayed wouldn't be.

"The fetus is no longer alive. The sack around the fetus is broken. We can wait for you to miscarry…" His words faded as my mind raced.

Wait! Miscarry? What? A numbness washed through me.

The doctor continued, "I think it would be best if we removed it. It would be very painful and messy to wait for it to abort itself and in the long run, best for you."

For me? What about my baby? God, stop calling it 'a fetus'! I wanted to scream, cry, hit something, and run. I wanted to turn back the hands of time and be anywhere but in that cold, sterile room with a doctor telling me that my *baby*—not my *fetus*—was dead.

But, I couldn't change anything. I agreed to the D & C (dilation and curettage), which is when the cervix is dilated and the fetal and placental tissues are scraped or suctioned out. I felt afraid and shocked. I couldn't believe the life inside of me was no longer alive. Just that feeling was beyond explanation. However, something inside triggered me to agree to remove the baby because I figured it would be worse to wait, day after day, for it to abort itself. I knew I couldn't handle that trauma, so I chose another.

I left in a state of disbelief. I couldn't even cry.

When my husband got home the next day, I told him the news. The day after that, I went in for my day surgery.

The doctor told me that upon examining the fetal tissue, he discovered it was "perfectly normal" and that first pregnancy miscarriages were very common. I swear he almost smiled, as if this was no big deal. I was young, and there'd be no problems in getting pregnant again.

Was that supposed to help? They were *common?* Maybe if I'd been told that there was a concrete reason for my miscarriage, i.e., an abnormality in the chromosomes or an infection that would render my baby ill, I'd have felt it was a blessing. Or, maybe not.

"Wait a few months and you can try again." the doctor said.

Try again? Let me get over this!

That was just the beginning of a very long, painful road I was about embark upon. One on which no one understood my grief. Why? Because there was no 'baby' to be seen. There was no real sense of loss for anyone but me. People cared, but more about me than my lost child. The child I carried and loved in my womb for four months. The child I had dreams and plans for. The child I talked to during the day.

The child that was never to be.

My Story
Dr. Linda Backman

Our first son, Joel, was born in December of 1969, following an easy conception, an uneventful, but filled with excitement and anticipation pregnancy, and a normal first delivery. Just as my naïve mind had expected, there were no major "hitches." When the time came approximately two years later to begin work on another pregnancy, I had no expectation of anything but a repeat experience. But if you have lived enough years of life to become more aware, you know that life is not always, in fact often it is not, a smooth path to the destination of your choice.

In the fall of 1971, I was pregnant for a second time. One afternoon during the tenth week of my pregnancy I discovered vaginal bleeding. Panic set in as I called a close friend, my doctor, and my husband who was out of town. The next sixteen weeks are a blur at this point. Numerous doctor visits continued with no clear explanation as to why I continued to bleed off and on, off and on, week after week. Ultrasound and sonograms were not being used in the early 1970s; therefore no medical means was available to ascertain from where the bleeding stemmed. Instructions changed week by week....bed rest, no bed rest, etc. Needless to say, managing life with a two-year-old son became rather complicated.

Week 26 of pregnancy arrived, and the bleeding increased. I was admitted to the maternity floor on a Friday. Each day through the weekend I recall talking to my baby and deeply wanting to believe, as I continued to feel movement, that he would be fine. On Monday contractions began, and I delivered a baby boy weighing slightly more than two pounds. Surreal is the only word to describe the experience. Our baby was born, they whisked him away, and what seemed like only a few minutes later (perhaps it was an hour) my doctor came to my husband and I and said, "Mrs. Backman, your baby has expired." Dr. S then turned and walked away.

Unbeknownst to me, grieving began immediately. In retrospect, it would be simple to suggest how people might have behaved differently and describe alternate behavior which might have assisted and facilitated my grieving. I came to understand that the general public and professional community had little understanding of how to support and guide me and my psyche.

Some thirty years hence, I now recognize the point where recognizable steps toward becoming a psychologist began, as I began to believe there were few, if any, people around me who knew what I needed emotionally and could explain my emotional ups and downs and nightmares. In particular, it is now crystal clear when and how life pointed me in the direction of teaching, guiding, and inspiring others to understand and allow grief to become transformative. No one intends to block the path to moving through grief, and, often, it is the 'hard way' that we come to know what we did need that was not happening.

With the knowledge I have today and with all the power in the world, I would have changed many parts of my experience with our second son, Adam. I place as much responsibility on my shoulders as anyone else's shoulders. Today, I would know more of what I needed and would be able to ask, but at twenty-five years of age speaking up just didn't occur. What would I have done differently?

I would have asked many more questions of the doctors during the long weeks of bleeding off and on. I would have come to understand what the possible explanations were, and what could be done, if anything. Much later I was given minimal detail and told the complication was unlikely to happen in the future. And, in fact, two years later I delivered a healthy daughter…what a thrill.

—*I would have held my baby, my child!*

—I would not have let the doctor just say my baby had expired without asking for further detail. Fortunately, our pediatrician at the time came to examine our baby and offered me details of what he found….bless him.

—I would not have agreed with my husband and parents going ahead and choosing a casket, planning a service, and carrying out the service at the cemetery without me. I was *so* young and naïve. Perhaps I will never understand why the rabbi involved went along with such a plan. What I do know is that the death/loss of a child scares people.

—I wouldn't have waited six years before placing a permanent marker on Adam's grave, giving him a first name formally, and creating our own family service.

And so many "I would haves" and "I wouldn't haves" continue, which is absolutely a part of life and learning.

I know in my heart of hearts that I was led to gain an understanding of the grief process, assist others in grief, and become a mental health professional broadening the scope of my ability to educate and help others. Perhaps, most importantly, I allowed the transformative process within to unfold and to guide me to this point in my life where I can write to you, the reader, and say you can get beyond this, and your life can magnify into its intended beauty.

But....you *must* walk the path, feel the feelings, and keep on moving forward with loving support around you. This is my wish for you.

Marnie's Story
Marnie Pehrson

It was an early summer morning as I walked down the church hallway in Chattanooga, Tennessee. One of my friends waved and asked me how I was feeling. I told her that I felt amazingly great—the best I'd felt in months. The nausea was gone, and it was almost like it had stopped overnight. Other than a strange twinge of pain I'd experienced on Friday (which I didn't mention to anyone), this pregnancy seemed to be rolling along fine, just as my last three had.

A couple days later I was in my OB/GYN's office for my first checkup. I was already sixteen weeks along, but considering myself an "old hand" at the pregnancy thing, I didn't rush in for my first checkup.

It's always a pleasurable experience to go into my doctor's office, not that I enjoy being poked or prodded, but my doctor has delivered all my babies and he's a caring physician and his nurses are kind and genuinely concerned women. Over the years, they've come to feel more like friends than medical professionals.

As Dixie put the monitor to my stomach and began searching for the heartbeat, she couldn't find one. I began to feel a bit uneasy, but Dixie assured me that sometimes babies can hide in there where she can't find a heart beat easily. She moved me to another room for my doctor to do an ultrasound. Again, no heartbeat, and my doctor began to brace me for the possibility that my baby was no longer alive. To be perfectly certain, it would require an internal ultrasound, and he sent me next door to the hospital. By now I was shaking and praying that surely this wasn't happening. I took a moment to call my husband at work and my parents to let them know what was happening and then made my way over to the hospital.

As I waited, my father appeared and sat down beside me, patting me on the knee and assuring me in his ever-loveable, calm, assuring manner that whatever happened, it would be for the best and that I would be fine. His presence was just what I needed to allay my fears and help me through the unbearable wait.

Finally they called me back to a tiny room filled so full of equipment that there was barely enough room for me and the technician to do the ultrasound. Again, no heartbeat. I returned to my doctor's office, and he told me they'd give me a week for my body to go into labor on its own. A long, empty week passed. It's a strange feeling carrying a baby inside you that you know is dead and waiting for labor pains to start that will bring you nothing of joy in the end.

Finally I was admitted to the hospital for the induction of labor. The nurses were wonderful. I asked my nurse if it were possible that they could just do one last ultrasound. Somehow I still clung to the possibility that my baby could be alive. Graciously, she assured me she understood, brought in an ultrasound machine, and performed one last scan. No miracle occurred; no infusion of life burst into my baby. The induction began. I'd had my first three babies naturally without drugs or epidurals, but this time my husband suggested that I take something. Why suffer needlessly? They gave me a mild pain killer, and it was a relatively painless experience.

When the baby finally emerged, he was ashen and gray. I asked the nurse to hold him up so I could see his little body. I remember he was bigger than I imagined he would be. I would have named him Samuel. They put me to sleep for a D & C. My husband stayed with me until night came, and then he went home to get some sleep. My mother cared for our other three children.

The next day in the hospital, I read, pondered, and prayed. I remember thinking how different you're treated after a miscarriage than a birth. It wasn't that I was treated poorly; I was just left alone. There was none of that coming in and checking on you every hour. I was left to think and ponder—which was exactly what I needed. While it was such a strange empty feeling and my arms ached to hold my baby, I felt a wonderful reassuring peace that all was as it should be. I believe that there are some souls who are simply too good for this world. While those of us living, learning, and growing on this earth are here to learn important lessons and be tested on them, there are others who are simply so perfect that they don't need this schoolroom we call mortality. They bypass this imperfect world or spend only a little time here and then return home to that perfect sphere from which our spirits come. My Samuel is one of these, and I feel honored to be his mother.

It was this faith and belief that brought me through an otherwise traumatic experience. The hardest part of it all was carrying our next child because of the underlying current of dread that what happened before could happen again. My doctor took special precautions to see that it did not, and on November 22, 1996, our healthy and beautiful daughter Jillian was born. Since that time, we've been blessed with two more sons. Many years later, our family still holds within our hearts a little boy we call Samuel whom we hope to meet again in a heavenly world.

Marnie Pehrson is the mother of 6. She and her family live in north Georgia where she works from home as an Internet developer and author. She is the founder of SheLovesGod.com and author of "Lord, Are You Sure?" and "The Patriot Wore Petticoats," among others. Read excerpts from her books at MarniePehrson.com.

Mary's Story
MaryBeth Foster

When Ellen asked me to write about my miscarriage, I had to stop and think. So much was going on at the time. I had just had a baby, and she wasn't even crawling around yet. Also, I still vividly remembered her birth, the pain, the fear. So, I think my story is a bit different than most. I think one of the reasons is I'm far too analytical, or so I've been told. I don't see that in myself.

I did a lot of reading when I was pregnant with my first child. One of the things I read was a small pamphlet on miscarriage. About the only thing it really said to me was that miscarriages generally happen due to the fact that there is something wrong with the fetus. I was satisfied with that knowledge.

When I miscarried, I still was experiencing the fear from my first birthing.

I've since had many more children and am the proud mother of five now, all natural births.

The day of the miscarriage is still vivid in my mind, as are the days after my miscarriage. I was at my mother's house—stuck there with my daughter. I was supposed to stay overnight.

I was cramping badly and knew deep down I was miscarrying. However, I didn't say anything right away. My mother (the expert) had had five miscarriages and five children.

I digress. I was there with my young daughter and my mother. We were playing with Elizabeth (my daughter), and the cramping became much more profound. After just having Elizabeth, I knew what those cramps were. So, I went upstairs to the bathroom and spent quite a long time on the toilet waiting for all of it to pass. I was about 6 weeks along—not far at all as far as pregnancy goes. However, I still knew I was losing a life. One that could have been much like the beautiful daughter I just had.

The mass finally passed. Somehow, I was able to relax and go back downstairs...

What I really wanted to do was go home, but, like I said, I was stuck there. Neither my other nor I drove. My father was at work and so was my husband (at the time).

I remember telling my mother that it hurt really bad and that I didn't feel well at all. What I got in return was a, "Knock it off; miscarrying isn't painful; get over it."

That was the end of that. I was very angry, to say the least, and never mentioned it again.

I went home the next day and called my doctor. I was seen right away. We confirmed that I had miscarried, and again, that was that.

But it wasn't the end of that. For the next week or three, I don't remember how long, my mother and everyone else kept saying: *It was for the best, It will be okay,* and *It's not that unusual to miscarry.* All I wanted to do was put that part of my life behind me and move on. I had a brand new baby daughter, and a new life to look forward to.

But, then I really thought about what Ellen asked me to write about, and I wasn't so sure I could do that. You see, analytically speaking, I accepted my miscarriage. I reasoned it was okay, actually convinced myself of it. But, it's not as cut and dry as that.

The more I think about it, the more I realize that it was almost like losing two, not one, birthed babies.

But, I guess that would be for a different story.

*A note from Ellen: Everyone deals with grief in their own way, and Mary's experience shows how difficult it can be when we turn to those closest to us for support, only to have our pain dismissed—as if it were nothing. It's critical that anyone around a woman who has miscarried, acknowledge her grief, let her feel it and deal with it as she may. To hear the words "get over it," especially from someone you love, hurts deeply. Although their intentions may be good (trying to get you away from a painful situation by forcing you to focus on other things), it isn't healthy in my opinion—and it hurts. I heard those very same words. I can attest to that.

Grieving

The day I got home from my D & C—or removal of the fetus—I was overcome with so many emotions that my head swam. Other than feeling sick from the procedure, I had to accept that I was no longer pregnant while my hormones still told me otherwise. I had to rid myself of dreams that would never be and face the fact that I'd never hold or see my baby.

That day, family members came by to see how I was holding up. They offered words of comfort. My husband watched me cry on the couch not knowing what to do. I was thankful for the caring but wanted to be left alone.

By the second day I was up and about. Still not feeling well by a long shot, at least I was off the couch. I'd go to the bathroom and burst into tears when I saw the blood that was still coming out of me. I'd pick up the one small outfit I bought for the baby and caress it gently, knowing that the small body I wanted desperately to fill it would never exist.

Life did go on, but I couldn't let go. I even was told once to, "Grow up and get over it."

I functioned, but I carried with me a sadness that went to my very core. There was no closure. The only closure I had was that somewhere in a hospital were the remains of my baby. No service. No funeral. Nothing. People don't do that for babies they haven't held.

But, what of babies that were loved more than anything? Because my baby wasn't seen I was supposed to pretend he or she didn't exist?

I couldn't.

I felt very alone in my grief. I didn't know (back then) that there were support groups for women who miscarried. I didn't have access to the Internet and all of its resources. I couldn't find any books telling me how to get on with my life after miscarrying.

Let me say this: Your grief is *very* real, and you are entitled and need to go through the process. You have suffered a tremendous loss and to deny yourself the chance to grieve serves only to prolong your agony. This is not something that can be tucked into the far recesses of your heart and mind. Why? Because it'll eat you up inside. You cannot move forward if you don't allow what's only natural. Cry if you want to. Feel your pain even if others don't find it necessary. If someone questions you and your grief, don't let them convince you that your ordeal is inconsequential. It isn't. I'm not recommending that you grieve forever—but, I am saying that it needs to be done. Allow yourself to feel!

Grieving
Dr. Linda Backman

Grief has become my specialty. Strange though it may sound, as a therapist I find great comfort and pleasure in working with someone who needs support and direction in moving through grief. Grief can be horribly frightening...we often think we are truly "losing our minds," losing our grip on reality and balance. The truth is we must, for a period of time, fall into the abyss of pain and grieve heavily. Our neat and clean American society has "whitewashed" grieving, suggesting we can move through significant loss in a month, or two, or three. Nothing could be any further from the truth.

About a week ago, I attended the ancient ritual in Jewish culture of completing the first year of mourning with the "unveiling" of my aunt's headstone. As my cousin explained during the service, traditionally Jews mourn for a period of eleven months following a death. Jewish law guides and normalizes acute grief as lasting at least eleven months. During this period of time the grieving individual recites the Kaddish mourner's prayer regularly and is viewed as being in a unique state or place of grief. How wise were Jews, along with numerous other ancient cultures, to sanction the behavior of someone in grief. It is absolutely normal and acceptable to focus on the death of your loved one for as much as a year or longer.

How clearly I recall coming home from the hospital three days after delivery without a baby in my belly and without a baby in my arms. Never have I felt so empty. How clearly I recall the friends and family who were there for me and acknowledged our loss. How clearly I recall the friends and family who seemed to avoid me. Today, I understand the fear people feel that death could "bite" anyone. Today, I understand the lack of information and education about death and grief, which would have assisted my friends and family in knowing how to approach me.

Grief is a process. Grief takes time...more time than you expect in the beginning. When you feel the most abnormal and out of control, you are truly the most normal. We must allow ourselves to feel the pain of grief. A wound must be allowed to hurt, to be exposed to the light of day, in order to heal. A wound does not heal if it is covered tightly and not allowed to breathe.

Grief is a series of stages, but not fluid step-by-step stages. Grief can't be characterized mathematically like two plus two plus two equals six. Grief is here, there, and everywhere, but once a year or more goes by you can look back and view the process. It is horribly chaotic seeming when you look ahead, but looking back over time we can see where we were going and that there is a purpose. At times, you must hang on for your life, because you will feel as if you are going to be swallowed whole. In oversimplified terms, the following is a list of normal stages/feelings you are quite likely to experience, not necessarily in a particular order:

Numbness/Disbelief/Fog
Crying
Could have done/Should have done
Someone or something is to blame
Anger
Depression
Physical symptoms
Insomnia
Withdrawal

You must have support in some form. It matters not the form. Support could be a spouse, a friend, a family member, a group, or a spiritual foundation, as long as that individual or group will allow you to chart your own course and be supportive at the same time. There is no specified course. At times, professional guidance is useful and perhaps necessary. *You have not failed* if you opt for therapy and/or medication. The key is to feel your feelings and know you are going through a normal process.

Grieving can be more difficult if you have suffered significant loss already in your life. When I speak of loss...I mean just that...loss of all sizes, shapes, and varieties. I am not referring to loss only through death. I am referring to loss through divorce, through difficult relationships, through illness....any manner of loss where you no longer have something or someone in your life who meant a great deal to you. Any type of loss which seems completely outside of what you might have expected to occur in your life. No one is made of stone, and no one is an island. We all have times when we crumble. We all have times when we need support from others. Weakness, to me, means we won't accept loving arms to catch us when we fall.

And what of transformation....can grieving guide us into a transformative space? If there is any purpose to loss, the purpose is, beyond a doubt, that of transformation or, essentially, altering our previously held view of life. If I had not, ultimately, come to this conclusion following the death of our second child, I would not be writing these words one by one. In many ways, the course of my life was altered dramatically with Adam's loss. Facing my feelings, coping with grief, took the steering wheel of life out of my hands and led me onto a new highway. I will never be the same, nor would I want to be. But, did I know this within a year or two of Adam's birth and death? Of course not.

Blame

Who could I blame for this? Did I do something wrong? Did that glass of wine I had before I even knew I was pregnant somehow hurt my baby? Did that slip on the ice have anything to do with it? What about the cigarettes I smoked? Or, or, or...

It's a very natural thing to blame yourself when you suffer a miscarriage. I did. I wracked my brain in a futile attempt to come up with some answers. *Anything.* Nothing the doctor said could convince me that there wasn't something I did to make this happen.

So, I prolonged my suffering. By blaming myself I only made things worse. It was not my fault—just as it's not your fault that you've miscarried. No, that glass of wine or beer you had did not cause your miscarriage. No, the argument you had with your husband did not cause you so much stress that you miscarried. No, the unhealthy food you ate from a fast food restaurant didn't do it either. Please, stop knocking yourself and blaming yourself for this. I know you need answers. You want some sort of justification for your pain and loss. But, when you continually find, or try to find blame within yourself, you are hurting yourself over and over again.

When I couldn't find blame within myself—or at least a concrete event that I could somehow link to my miscarriage, my anger turned to God. Yes, God. How could He let this happen? Why? What did I do to deserve this?

I never thought about the bigger plan. Back then, my views on life and what God's plans were for me were much different. Even if they weren't, I still would have felt tremendous pain, and my faith would have been tested to the max. I still would have wondered what kind of a God would allow such a thing to happen.

Over time, however, I learned to stop blaming God. I don't want to preach to you, but, to those of you who are looking to God for answers, you'll probably never know. In retrospect, I can now look back and realize that it was all a part of the plan for my life and accept that, as painful as it may be. It certainly isn't something I'd want to relive, and

I still don't know why it happened. My marriage did end. Maybe that's part of it. Maybe my ex-husband and I just weren't cut out to be parents—we weren't cut out to be married. But, that doesn't apply to everyone, and I'm only using examples pulled from my own life. There are many women who aren't involved with partners but have miscarried. Many women have terrific marriages and miscarry. You all have your own circumstances to look at and to try to find blame in. Let me just say this: Please, for your own peace of mind, stop blaming yourself and God (if you're blaming Him, too). It's simply torture, and the more you search for answers, the longer you prolong your misery. I know it hurts. I can feel your pain. I know having the answers would take away a little of your pain. But, please consider this: Even if you had the answer right in front of you, would it really lessen your grief or sadness?

I know it wouldn't have with me. It wouldn't bring back what I lost. I know that now—only after time.

Acknowledge your pain. Feel it. But, please stop blaming yourself, God, or anyone else.

Blame
Dr. Linda Backman

Blame...what a complicated word. For most of us, when things go awry in our life we seek to find a place of blame, for we are seeking to gain *control* in our life. As the course of living proceeds, generally somewhere between the ages of twenty-five and thirty, we are hit with the not-so-gentle reality of life having its own plan. How many times have we as adults tried to avoid the small child or even teen walking or driving and paying no attention to anything but where they are going? This is the stage of life we often refer to as *invincible,* where we never even consider we can't do or have just what we choose.

As you are reading this book your next response might be, "Wrong!" You, just like Ellen and I, have had that cold blast of harsh reality bite you and force you, not so gently, to recognize we don't just decide to have a child, get pregnant, and live happily ever after.

So, who or what or where can we blame for the intensely painful loss of our wished-for child? Ellen has shared with you the typical course of blame where we seek to "beat-up" on ourselves, God, and elsewhere struggling to find an answer to why our baby died. I won't till the same ground, but want to share with you what is normal during grieving. In addition, I will be sharing my notion of transformation that can happen as we grieve.

First and foremost, blame and guilt are usual steps we walk during grief. Experiencing the struggle, the search for where to lay your frustration/anger over this loss is part and parcel of mourning. The key is not whether you blame someone or something, but whether you get stuck in this mode. Stuck means stuck for a significant length of time, months to years. A firm gauge is difficult if not impossible to ascertain. If you question whether you are truly imbedded in your blame, consult someone with professional training. Let me say one more time, if you are seeking to place blame within the first six months to a year of grieving, you are likely in a very normal stage.

I believe the truth is we seek to place blame, but are truly upset, and, perhaps, angry because our child is gone. Talking to your child and saying that you miss him/her is perfectly normal. Saying you would have wished or begged for a different outcome is also well within normal limits. Not having this child in your arms is the core of why we blame and feel guilt. If you can own these as your feelings you are likely to lessen the need to focus your loss elsewhere.

One's spouse is an extremely common focus for the pain of grief. A relationship with a solid foundation, generally doesn't crumble under the strain of grief. If your relationship has suffered lack of solidity for some length of time, projecting your pain and grief onto your partner can be highly risky. Once again, seek some professional guidance if you feel the need.

Let me continue to remind you that grief is a "roller coaster process." Please expect to feel solid one moment and completely disjointed the next. Some say grief is like standing in the ocean and having a wave come from behind causing you to fall face forward into the water. Keep on feeling and feeling and feeling…talking and talking and talking…as you knead the dough so will it rise.

In my opinion, when you begin to sense there must be some purpose for this loss you are truly moving forward. Nothing will remove the pain…but recognizing there is some purposeful alteration in your life, which stemmed from the death of your child, can offer you a deeper perspective. Without a grasp on what lies beyond the excruciating pain, you are likely to get caught in the spider web of why. *But*…a greater perspective often is not to be had in the first few months to a year of grief. Please be patient with yourself…this too shall pass into clarity.

Allow me to recount a quick story, if I may. Our child who died was our second son, who was two years younger than our first. Two years after the birth and death of Adam, our daughter was born. My pregnancy and delivery were quite normal. Eighteen years later, when our daughter went off to college, she met a young man who later became her husband and our son-in-law. This new man in our family is almost exactly the same age as Adam would have been and has many physical and personality similarities to our oldest son. We have always felt very comfortable with him. Doesn't life hand us some very odd twists?

Letting Go

This is probably the most challenging thing I had to do after my miscarriage. To this day I'm still affected by it. I still feel twinges of pain when I see mothers walking their babies. I sometimes get teary when walking past the newborn section in a department store. I've gone to baby showers and found myself having to 'step out for some air,' not being able to embrace the joy. The memories of my miscarriage still sneak up on me—out of the blue—and the pain bursts towards the surface of my heart.

That's what I meant earlier when I said, "I've never *forgotten* my miscarriage." It's like anything painful in your life—any loss or trauma that you've experienced. There are certain things that trigger the emotions to come back. Sometimes, you can't figure out what did it. It doesn't have to be as obvious as a baby shower or seeing a mother with her child. It can just happen. When it does, allow yourself to feel. Burying it will serve no other purpose other than hurting you. It's your mind and spirit's way of saying, "I need to let go of this feeling right now and the only way I can do so is to *allow myself to feel it."*

It's all part of the process of letting go.

Please don't think of it as a setback. I used to. Months or even years after my miscarriage, I'd find myself crying over it. I still do. Something would happen deep inside of me, and it was like living it all over again. The pain was just as real. The loss was just as deep.

If I didn't allow myself to 'let it out,' where would those feelings have gone? Each time you deny yourself the experience of feeling—even if it's sadness—you're putting an obstacle in your road to moving on. The more obstacles, the more difficult it is to go forward.

Just as you can't blame yourself for your miscarriage, you can't blame yourself for being human and feeling. Please don't confuse your feelings with an inability to move on with your life. It's all part of moving on, and you simply can't do it if you continually block your own path by holding everything in.

When you need to 'clear your road of obstacles' so that you can move on, do it. You're entitled, and it's normal.

Think of it like this: If any of you have lost a parent, a pet, or someone close to you, don't you still feel sad sometimes over it? Do you have yourself a good cry—even if it's been months or years since it happened? After you cry or 'let it out,' do you feel a sense of release? Why, then, is this not the same?

Letting go takes a long time. At least it did for me. I define 'letting go' like this: I've not forgotten that my miscarriage happened; I still feel the pain sometimes, and I allow myself to. But, I've stopped blaming myself or anyone else for it and have accepted, although painfully, that it's a part of my life that I cannot change. I am not bitter at the world anymore, and I am now moving on down the road of my life, open to new experiences.

Letting Go

Dr. Linda Backman

Will we 'move on' if we don't allow ourselves to 'let go'? My honest opinion is "No." Will we forget our child if we let go? Once again, the answer undeniably is "No." Can we control our feelings forever...not allowing pain to be felt? Or in an opposite manner, do we need to feel difficult feelings, ad nauseam, for months and years in order to honor and remember our child? No, no, and once again, no!

The process of grieving is to Let Go on a regular basis in order to allow what is natural. Feelings are as normal as apple pie, but we are taught to hold them inside causing further distress. And for goodness sake, please don't buy into the words we often hear as children from our unknowing parents who say, "You made me angry when you did..." We don't *make* anyone feel anything. Others do not make us feel poorly...and the reverse is also the case. Our feelings are our feelings...not created by anyone else.

How well I remember a day somewhere near Adam's First Anniversary when I said to myself, "It is time to stop feeling so much pain so much of the time. Will it do me or Adam any good to go on feeling such agony? I am so tired of not living my life. I *must* break out of this constant spiraling downward." My son needed me, my husband needed me, but more importantly, I needed me.

In the grieving process we must put one foot in the front of the other. There are days and periods of time where these steps are definitely very mini-steps. Don't be shocked if, at times, you believe you have slid all the way back to the beginning. The overall picture is the key. Do you move ahead either more quickly or farther forward after the fall? It is not bad...you are not bad when feelings overwhelm you. I can't scream loud enough, "You are normal!" Grief is, as I have said, the time in your life when you feel 'all over the map.'

But...there comes a time after months and months of grief, where we must evaluate: Where we are? Have you had many more miserable days than good ones for many, many months or more than a year? If so, it is, more than likely, the point in time to 'pull yourself up by those bootstraps' and move forward in your life. For some, feeling absolutely stuck is the signal to join a grief support group and/or seek a psychotherapist skilled in matters of bereavement. It is no crime whatsoever to need some additional support. The loss of a loved one, in this case the loss of your child, can be the most devastating emotional experience life has ever handed to you. Remember when you have a child die, you have not only lost someone in your life, but you have also lost a future you had anticipated.

Letting go is often surprisingly difficult. If you have grieved for many months or years, you have set a pattern of 'the glass half empty' relative to how your daily living happens. In order to transform your life into 'the glass half full' you may need to force some alteration in your routine. For instance, if you have done nothing but go to work and come home since your pregnancy loss, it may be necessary to literally schedule new activities. For example, find a capable massage therapist in your area and book a regular appointment. Ask a friend to plan an afternoon or evening out once each week. Join an exercise class that meets two or three times per week. Once the new plan is in place, deleting a 'for you' item off your schedule is just not allowed...if you don't take care of you it won't happen.

I want to reiterate: The most common fear in letting go is that your baby will be forgotten. This will simply not happen. In my mind it is completely impossible. Certain experiences in life are written indelibly onto our heart and spirit. And such experiences are profound teachers. I would hazard to say that each and every one of us who has walked the journey of pregnancy loss has found life permanently transformed. What was crucial or important before no longer seems to rank high on the priority list. Other much more significant endeavors have evolved into the critical matters and ways we spend our time. For this be thankful, for you have become a much more sensitive, concerned, and caring individual.

Many of us following pregnancy loss now devote our life and our energy to projects and concerns which greatly assist the world in some obvious ways...and also in some not so obvious, but equally important ways. It matters not how your life changes, it only matters that you have factored your loss into the fabric of your life. For, without such transformation, your loss, in my mind, has not created the 'birthmark' it might have.

Moving On

None of us knows what life has in store for us. There are going to be great, beautiful things happening, and there are going to be painful things that try your spirit. Accepting the challenge, or 'moving on,' is what life's about.

I know that as painful as my miscarriage was for me, it served a purpose in my life. I'm not saying that this is a good thing to have happen to you! What I mean is that without that terrible event, I would not be able to write these words in the hope of helping you. If I hadn't lived it, I couldn't talk about it like this. If I didn't cry the tears that you've cried, you wouldn't give a hoot about what I'm saying to you.

Why would you? What would I know of your grief, sadness, blame, guilt, and fear?

I do know.

There are so many of us on different paths. We are professionals in the workforce or professional mothers. We are painters and singers. We are caretakers, and we are movie stars. Some of us may have children, while some of us don't. My point is that we all have our own lives, and our diversity is wonderful. The one thing that connects us all is that we are women who experienced a terrible loss that seemed, in many cases, to go unacknowledged by many. We have all felt the dismissal of our very real grief, and we have all felt alone and isolated because of it. We have all wondered what 'might have been,' and we have all been caught off guard by powerful emotions resurfacing.

As you move on down your road, whatever that road may be, I want you to know that what you're experiencing is something that I, along with millions of other women, have experienced. This does not lessen your pain—it *acknowledges* it. You are not abnormal for crying 'too much.' You are not going crazy when years have passed and you still find yourself remembering and feeling. We cry our tears together. You are not alone in your struggle to get through this...

Most importantly, you will.

Moving On
Dr. Linda Backman

Moving on may seem a complete impossibility as you attempt to navigate your way through the grief process. Nonetheless, time and honestly experiencing and labeling your feelings will allow you to arrive at the point where life becomes tolerable, meaningful, and, even, pleasant once again. Frequently, perhaps most of the time, the recognition of having progressed into some degree of happiness occurs as we glance over our shoulder. It seems most of us can only risk a retrospective view of our emotional state once a sufficient decrease in the pain of loss has been felt. During the depths of grief it is an impossible task to gain a 'bird's eye view' of ourselves in order to recognize where we dove into the river of loss and how close to the other shore we may or may not be. Believe it or not, we do ultimately find life to be, once again, worth living.

You have traveled upon a long and arduous journey. Congratulate yourself for having summited the highest mountain in your world. You made it by just taking one step at a time and no more. This alone is to be applauded, for grief, at times, can seem like quicksand. Each forward step can require immense fortitude in order to avoid the 'stuckness' or permanence of paralyzing pain.

Those of us who have survived the loss of a child and become friends of the resulting transformation know our feet have plodded through those moments of 'this pain will never ever end.' But, somehow, by feeling all we can feel and having support around us, we discover that the texture of life looks, feels, and tastes radically different than before. Can we describe or explain the resulting alteration in how our worldview has been redirected? As a mother of a child lost prior to viability, I cannot fully define how Adam's death led me to take a particular exit off the freeway I was following at age twenty-five.

If I had to label my old highway it would be called "Interstate Sleepwalk," where I simply moved from day to day with no sense of a deeper process underlying my life. And, more so, I thought I knew what was truly important. Over the last thirty years my life has followed a very different path from what I thought was my destiny. Becoming a psychologist with an ongoing psychotherapy and healing practice was triggered by Adam's death. Becoming deeply involved with issues surrounding death and grief and spirituality have stemmed from my need to understand the deeper meaning of the loss of our second child. In addition, I have sought to gain a more profound respect for what life has to offer that we neither expect nor seek.

Experiencing the ending of a much wanted pregnancy and child is phenomenally difficult, but I know it has carved its mark into my life and soul. For this, in some odd and strange way, I am grateful. I am a much more sensitive, attuned individual than I might ever have been. For me, with thankfulness, there was a child who came after and stayed. Parenting her, I believe, has been dramatically affected by having Adam die. My professional work is deeply and profoundly tied to the knowledge that the Universe knows better than we what is necessary in the tapestry of our life. I truly believe accepting the lack of power and control we have in our life is fundamentally important. If there were no ups and downs in life we would have neither respect nor understanding of the mystery of each step along life's route. I speak of the concept "If X had not happened, would Y or Z have followed in sequence?

Once again, let me remind you of what I call the 'nose against the glass' theory. When we are deep in grief it is absolutely impossible to step back from our feelings in order to cope. This is what happens to everyone. Furthermore, we have not a shred of perspective in life. We simply know we hurt like—well, you understand. What I can offer you is trust: trust that if you keep on feeling, crying, and asking for support you will ultimately succeed in arriving at the point of Moving On. Will all your pain be gone? The answer is "No." Will you forget your loss completely? The answer is "No."

You will find life continues and you are no longer the same person you were prior to the loss of your child. Surviving pregnancy loss can and does happen.

My Angel Baby

When I found out you were there—
growing inside of me,
I was surprised and a little scared—
of how our life would be.

But, I loved you from the moment—
I knew that you were there.
Even though we hadn't planned you—
I felt joy beyond compare.

And then one day I noticed—
that I did not feel right.
My sister to my rescue—
to save me from this plight.

A cold and sterile table—
I sat upon in fear.
The doctor looked for you—
and found that you weren't there.

God wanted you my little one—
not on this earthly plane.
Not a day has passed my dear one—
that I haven't felt the pain.

He said you weren't "viable."
I asked, "What does that mean?"
He replied you were not living—
and my heart began to scream.

For sixteen weeks I had you—
warm within my womb.
And although I'll never know you—
My love's as constant as the moon.

My arms will never hold you,
your eyes I will not see—
I'll never feel you sleeping
so softly upon me.

Sometimes there are no answers
to the tragedies in life.
I must believe that God—
knew the moment wasn't right.

So much time has passed—
since that empty, lonely time.
But even as I write this,
my eyes with tears do shine.

But please remember precious one—
in Heaven up above—
You'll always be my Angel Baby—
You'll always have my Love.

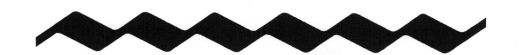

Part Two

Miscarriage Fallout

Over the many years since I miscarried, I discovered ways to help me heal as time marched on. When the pain of miscarriage and subsequent 'fallout' occurred, I searched for ways to help me cope, breath, relax, live! I was desperate to find tools which would calm my racing body, release my overactive mind, help dry the tears. In addition, my anxiety attacks were triggered after my miscarriage, so I dove head-first to find something to make them subside as they were nearly debilitating. As you read through Part Two of this book, please understand that everything may not apply to you. If it feels right, incorporate a relaxation tool or technique into your life—making it your own. If it doesn't, don't force it. We are all different, experience pain differently, and our journey to healing and recovery after miscarriage requires different helpers, if you will. What's important to me is that you find something, even if only one thing, to assist you as you travel the often rocky, but very worthwhile path towards resuming a quality life.

Miscarriage fallout—what a term, but I think it's the best way to sum up what I felt after my miscarriage, and probably what you're feeling. The are so many emotions, thoughts, shattered dreams and wishes that accompany a miscarriage—fallout seemed the best word. The dreams of pregnancy, your baby, what life will be like with your new baby, and the anticipation of the baby's arrival...are gone. That's a tough adjustment to make. Those very things make some days nearly impossible to get through without constantly holding your tears back, afraid you'll burst at any moment. That's what these tools are for—those days when you feel yourself slipping, depressed, wound up, and anxious. I lived many days that way after my miscarriage, and quite frankly, I still have days like that. It all depends what life throws our way. The tools and techniques shared with you on the following pages are meant to slow you down, calm you down—placing you on a brighter, easier path. I use these tools today, whenever I need a pick-me-up or a thought adjustment. So, they apply to your life now and throughout your life because part of life is stress. How we cope is key to getting through it successfully with the least damage done.

Writing this book sometimes brings up painful emotions. It's only natural that in writing about miscarriage and ways to heal and cope, triggers to my own painful experiences go off like shots in the night. When that happens, I have to step away, regroup, and begin again. How? I use what I'm going to share with you. These relaxation and stress reduction techniques work, and I've given them a fifteen-year trial run.

To give you an example, I was writing the other day and felt completely blocked. I couldn't place my finger on why, but was all too familiar with the feelings bubbling up inside. My breathing was shallow. I felt restless, anxious, and the more I waited, the worse it got. I found myself wanting to cry and knew I needed to give my mind a break. After all, I'm only human, and for as far as I've come, I still feel. It's like anything in life that leaves a scar. You move on and grow, but certain things trigger feelings associated with any painful event, in this case, miscarriage. Sometimes it's only for a moment or two and I'm fine. When it's more than a moment or two, I know it's time to practice some of the methods mentioned here to calm myself down, clear my mind, feel what I need to, and begin again. I believe it's a cycle we go through many times in this life. That's the part that's tricky. I'm sharing helpful tools, hoping to get you through some rocky days, when my own rocky days were the catalyst for learning these techniques.

After I miscarried, I barely got through a day without crying—and that lasted for a long time. So long, I wondered if I was going crazy because I just couldn't shake the feelings inside. It got to the point where I couldn't walk past baby food in a grocery store or baby clothes in a department store without feeling like I was going to burst. What a number it did on my mind and body. I was wound up like a top. Perhaps you feel the same way.

Fifteen years later, there are moments when I look at mothers walking their babies and feel pangs of emotion creeping to the surface. I remember how I felt after I miscarried like it was yesterday, and all the what-ifs start to play in my mind like a tape stuck on play. However, fifteen years ago I didn't have the advantage of knowing how to better deal with my feelings. Today, I've got ways to get myself through painful memories or events. Life throws us some pretty tough curve balls, along with the beautiful blessings. It's the curve balls I'll help take the curve out of, and the blessings will hopefully be seen more clearly.

As you can probably see, the tools in this part of the book were born out of a need. That need was created after my miscarriage, and during other stressful events. I say this because as grateful as I am for the wonderful blessings I've received, I know that life doesn't always go according to plan, and there are times when I use the tools mentioned here again, and again, and again.

Many have become a part of my daily life. Not all of them at once, of course. But, when I find myself getting wound up by something as trivial as a traffic jam, there are techniques I use to calm down. What good does it do me, or you for that matter, to get anxious or upset over waiting in traffic? None. It's not going to make the cars move any faster. It'll only make your insides race faster. Not good.

When you're ready to pick up this book and begin exploring ways to settle yourself down and gain a clearer perspective of what it is you're feeling and how to calm down when your feelings get the best of you, it's here. I'm here. I'm offering suggestions to help get you through a particularly rough moment, day, week, or more because I owe it to you. We are sisters bound by a common thread: miscarriage. And, for as lost as I felt after I miscarried, I want to offer you something I simply couldn't find: tangible hope. Someone telling you time heals everything and life will go on, may be correct but you already know that, and quite frankly, it doesn't *help*. The suggestions to aid you in your recovery are substantial, easy, don't require much attention span, and they'll smooth out the seas when they get too rough. There are ways to cope better as you heal, the two being entirely different. We can look at healing as the process of a wound, in this case, the trauma left behind after your miscarriage, closing up and *healing* over time. Yes, there may be a scar. But, the wound will not always be open, raw, exposed, and painful. Coping is how you *handle life* while your wound is healing. Coping is key to simply getting through the day—through anything that presents a challenge or a test to your spirit.

I hope you find something within the pages of this section to help you during other stressful times in your life. We all know they're bound to happen, and when they do, it's best to be prepared with all the backup you can get.

Onward we go. Let's explore the power of the positive, thoughts to ponder, anxiety, Reiki, relaxation, exercise, creativity, and journaling.

With each word you read, remember: there's a real person behind them, who has lived what you're living, and who understands and supports you very much.

God bless you on your way.

Tools to Aid You on Your Road to Recovery

The Power of Positive Affirmations— Accentuate the Positive

There is tremendous power in your words and thoughts. Repeating negative things to yourself serves only one purpose: harm. It's so easy to fall into the negative thinking trap, especially after you've miscarried or suffered any kind of loss or hardship. The positive aspects of life become nearly invisible—to your eyes. They are still there, and it's during the most difficult and stressful times of your life that you must force yourself to remember them. It's not easy, but it's necessary. How? By forcing your mind to think positive thoughts, often times repeating them aloud to reinforce their messages. It may sound foolish, or feel awkward, but drastic times call for drastic measures. If you feel trapped in a ditch of negativity, it may be time to take a look at the way you think. Until I examined my thoughts, I was unaware of just how negative and self-destructive I was being. After my miscarriage I could think of nothing but the pain, the dreams that were gone, the baby that was never to be. I was lost within my grief, and my mind became used to repeating things like, "I'll never feel normal again. I'll never hold my baby. God, why did this happen to me? How come she's pregnant and I'm not?" Over and over, I repeated these things, until I lived it, breathed it, dreamed it. I no longer felt or saw any of the happiness life had to offer. As real as your grief is, there is another side of your life that lives on, a much happier side full of possibility. Reminding yourself of its existence will enable you to see the world as a brighter place, with hope shining through the fog. Eventually, you'll smile again, even amidst your grieving process.

For years, I've used positive affirmations—statements said either aloud or to yourself—that reinforce only positive messages. You may be wondering how you could possibly think positively now, and I don't blame you. However, now is the time when you need positive *anything* more than ever. I never turned to positive affirmations when my life was great and the seas were calm. Why would I? Using positive affirmations came out of a need to shed light upon the dark, scary fog I felt trapped in and surrounded by following the days, weeks, and months after I miscarried. Positive affirmations probably won't make you hop, skip, jump, and sing your way through the day. The only time I've ever seen that is in a musical. When life's got you by the throat, and you no longer see or believe there's a silver lining to every cloud, the power of positive thoughts and words is amazing. Right now you may be nodding your head, thinking, "No way. I don't buy it." Please stick with me and allow me to show you a couple of simple examples of positive versus negative thoughts and the impact they have on your perception of life.

You wake up in the morning and the very first thought you have is, "This day's going to stink. I don't even want to get out of bed." But, you do, and as you make your way to the kitchen for some coffee or tea, your mind, being the clever thing it is, keeps repeating this message over and over, like a tape playing. You grab your coffee, get the kids fed, whatever—and your subconscious mind is still playing that tape, "This day's going to stink." Meanwhile, you're feeling more edgy, negative, sad, depressed—a wealth of emotions, none of which are good. You then go through the rest of the day like that, either at home or work. Perhaps you talk to a girlfriend on the phone and when she asks how you're doing, you tell her you've had a lousy day. It really stunk.

Beginning in the morning when you first opened your eyes, your brain told you your day was going to stink, and you believed it. Because you believed it, and repeated it, it actually manifested itself.

If that sounds a little hard to buy, let me flip the situation around. Apply all the examples from the first scenario to this one, with one major difference: When you open your eyes in the morning and your brain starts to tell you your day's going to stink, you immediately interrupt that thought pattern and say out loud, "Today is a new day. It's full of promise and hope. I'm open to good things coming my way, and I attract good things like a magnet." You then go through the rest of the day with *that* tape playing in your head.

Wow! Just reading the two examples of positive versus negative thinking gave me a shake! I've been in the 'this day's going to stink' mode many times before, so reading it was like another wake-up call. I've seen the difference beginning my day with a positive affirmation can make, and how repeating it throughout the day only serves to strengthen me, and ultimately, makes my days better.

Your brain is amazing, complicated, and mysterious. Your mind is even more so. Funny thing is, your body believes what your brain and mind tell it to. For example: If you tell yourself often enough that you're scared, depressed, hopeless, and/or tired, guess what? You will be. Have you ever done that? I know I have. I've even made very real situations worse. If I had a toothache and did nothing but think about and repeat how much it hurt, I made it hurt more because it's all I was focusing on. If I thought about the small bit of nausea I had, but told everyone I felt really sick, I ended up feeling really sick!

I wonder why it's so much easier for you, me—seemingly everyone, to be more negative than positive. I wish I had the answer. I can only say that thinking negative thoughts and repeating them over and over again turned me into a person I didn't recognize anymore. Where was the woman who always looked at the cup as being half-full? Where did I go? Where was the Ellen who always saw the good in people, counted her blessings, and no matter what life dished out, was able to see the light at the end of the tunnel?

I lost myself, and much of my strength, by unknowingly repeating negative messages to myself. It's so natural to do when life gets rough, and I wasn't even aware I was doing it. Who is? Does the average person give much thought to the way they're thinking—to the actual process of thinking?

Also, you're human, and all the positive affirmations in the world are not meant to deny you your feelings. If you're sad, you've every right to be sad. However, making it worse for yourself by reinforcing your sadness only serves to place a huge mountain smack dab in the middle of your road towards healing and recovery. No good ever comes from perpetually thinking negatively. I want to make the mountain on your road smaller or disappear entirely. That's not to say there's no healing process to go through. Of course there is. You don't need your brain making it harder to get through. Your brain and mind must be your allies, not your enemy.

If you're still not sold on the power of thought, that's your right. Let me share this with you: I once heard or read something that said, "Just imagine if everyone in the world thought nothing but positive thoughts at the same time." That really hit home with me. If that happened, the entire world would change, if only for a moment! If someone's thinking positive thoughts, they don't fight. When you're repeating loving, positive statements to yourself, you don't wage war, cry, hurt yourself or others. Talk about Utopia. Flip it around: Everyone's thinking negative, bad or evil thoughts at the same time. Scary! The world would be in worse shape than it already is. I can't even imagine the depths of destruction that would take place, and don't want to.

After I miscarried, I was a walking, talking, twenty-four-hour tape of negative thinking. So, what made me seek out positive affirmations? I didn't. They found me.

I spent a lot of time in bookstores after I miscarried, trying to find something to make me able to cope better. One day I was in a bookstore and something about a particular book drew me to it. It wasn't in with the grief and loss books, which is where I usually searched for help. I picked up the book, glanced at the title, and that alone struck a chord deep within me. *The Wisdom of Florence Scovel Shinn*—four of her complete works rolled into one book. I had no clue who this woman was, what she wrote of, but I knew I had to buy the book. So, I did.

That book forever changed the way I think. I still slip up and go on 'negative binges,' but when I do, her words burst forth, and I know I've got a chance at beating down the negative, replacing it with positive. I believe beyond a shadow of a doubt that my words and thoughts create my reality. That's not to say your miscarriage and the terrible ways you feel are not real—they are. But, you can either bury yourself in so deep you can't seem to dig yourself out, or you can *re-train your brain* to help you when the going gets really rough. I chose the latter, only after I realized I could.

Once the knowledge of positive thinking and its power was implanted in my mind, it was there for good. On my worst days, when life seems like it can't get any worse, my mind goes into auto-pilot and begins to soothe me with words of a positive nature. Sometimes, I feel like I'd rather drown in my own pity, but my mind simply won't allow it—at least not for very long.

I believe it's called self-preservation.

Thus began a new, uncharted course for me. After finding and reading that book, I began to change the way I thought because I knew I had to. My other option was to remain stuck in a place I didn't want to be in for the rest of my life—a very dark, scary, and lonely place. That scared me more than trying to change my way of thinking. I couldn't stay where I was. No way.

I can't possibly write affirmations with the eloquence of the late Florence Scovel Shinn, but I have written some that have helped me, and hopefully you'll find one or two that'll help you. If you do find one, you may want to write it down on a small card or piece of paper and stick it in your pocketbook or on your bathroom mirror. That way, as you begin the new journey of retraining your brain, you'll have a reminder right in front of you when your mind thinks it can get away with telling you your day's going to stink. Just say aloud something good—fifty times if you have to, and tell that negative thought to *go away, let me live today!*

Positive Affirmations

Allow— Today I allow myself to feel good things. I am not a bad person for feeling good. I will smile if I want to, laugh if I want to. Today I will feel good things.

Believe— I believe today is a new day full of hope, healing, and light. I am open to all that heals me and never lose sight of hope. I heal more with each moment.

Choose—Today I choose to be happy, joyful, and true to myself. The choice is mine. I choose happiness.

Doorway— The doorway to joy and healing is wide open. I step through the doorway of joy and healing, and slam the door on negative thoughts.

Each— Each day is a new day. Yesterday is gone. Today, I live in the *now* and see the beauty and good that surround me.

Faith— My faith in God, The Divine, A Universal Power, washes through me, ridding me of all my fears.

Give— What I give I will receive. When I give love, I get love. Today, I will give love.

God— God loves me, protects me, guides me, and heals me. Today, I walk with God. I thank God for loving me.

Hope— Hope surrounds me like a warm blanket. I walk through this day with the blanket of hope around me.

I— I am loved unconditionally by God. God's love lives within me and gets me through anything. I thank God for His love.

Jammed— The door to negative thinking is jammed shut! Today, only positive thoughts flow through me.

51

Kindness— I am kind and gentle to myself today. I am forgiving of myself today.

Love— The love of God reaches into every part of me and heals all my wounds.

My— My tears are dried by the loving hands of angels and replaced with comfort.

Negative— Negative thoughts create negative results. Today, I am positive and create positive results. I attract positive things into my life.

Open— Today I am open to God's plan for me. I trust God's plan.

Pray— Today I pray for healing and happiness. I believe I am receiving as I pray. I thank God for my healing and happiness.

Question— There is no question I am loved and cared for by God. There is no question God's love will get me through anything. God gives me the strength of a lion. I thank God for my strength.

Rest— Today is a day of rest for me. Rest comes easily and naturally. I am able to rest today.

Surrounded— I am surrounded by angels today. With each step I take, the angels are with me. The angels protect me, guide me, and comfort me. I offer thanks to the angels.

Thank— Today I thank God for all of my blessings. I see them clearly, and new blessings flow to me.

Understanding— Today I treat myself with the same understanding I give those I love. I am understanding and patient with myself.

Vanish— Doubt and fear vanish from my life today and are replaced with hope and faith!

With— With God, anything is possible. With God, *anything* is possible.

X— X marks the spot to my heart. God lives within my heart, and I take great comfort in that.

Yes— I say yes to all that is good! Goodness is attracted to me like a magnet!

Zest— Today I live zestfully. My spirit soars, I see my goals,and I will achieve them with zest!

Dial "A" for Anxiety Assistance

Anxiety is a natural human emotion. All of us experience anxious situations and without some anxiety, we wouldn't function properly. We need anxiety to get us out of dangerous situations. However, anxiety attacks are quite different, and very scary— especially the first time around. After any traumatic event, in this case a miscarriage, you may feel things inside of your body that scare you very much. Your heart may race for no reason, or your breathing may become very shallow. Women suffer from anxiety attacks more than men, but men get them, too. The thing is this: if you're really feeling like your body is acting out of control and it's terrifying you, please see your doctor. Don't do what I did and live with it for years before seeking help. There's nothing 'wrong' with you, it's just your body's way of saying, "I've had enough of this stress. I need to release it, and I'll do it with some adrenaline." There's help, hope, and healing.

For those of you who are ready to blow past this chapter because you don't suffer from anxiety, let me say this: I don't suspect that everyone reading this actually suffers from an anxiety disorder like I do. I'll bet many of you don't. If you do, you'll find help and reassurance. If you don't, you'll find help and reassurance. For purposes of this book, I don't want to equate anxiety with anxiety attacks, panic disorders, or any chronic, acute anxiety condition. Let's, for purposes of this book, define anxiety as a natural, human feeling of edginess and stress— because that's exactly what it is, and we all have it. Quite possibly, it's gotten to the point where it's inhibiting your life, or at least becoming a very unwelcome guest. To feel anxious at times is perfectly normal. We're wired that way. You're late for an appointment— you're anxious. You've got a doctor's appointment—you're anxious. You need to ace a test—you're anxious. It's a very normal feeling, and without it, we wouldn't function nearly as well as we do because anxiety, in the right 'doses'— gives us the extra push we need to perform at our peak. Notice I used the term 'doses.' When you're really stressed, depressed, etc., you can easily suffer from an anxiety overdose. And, let's face it, miscarriage is more than stressful. If you feel very anxious, it's no wonder. Don't beat yourself up for it, rather, try to understand it. That's what this chapter will do, and it'll help you get through those periods when you feel like you're about to tear your hair out or crawl out of your skin. Believe me, *I know.*

Stressful events make us anxious; it's as simple as that. Compound that with the grief, loss, sadness, etc., after a miscarriage, and you've got the unwanted recipe for high anxiety.

Don't mistake me for an anxiety expert, but I've dealt anxiety attacks for nearly eighteen years, if that counts for anything. During that period, I've learned a lot—about myself, the triggers to my anxious feelings, and most importantly, how to ease the uncomfortable bouts of anxiety into something a bit more manageable. I'm not promising to make them go away—I've yet to master that myself. That's not the point, nor do I know if it's entirely possible. However, let's focus on what I know: There are ways to make yourself more comfortable when you're stuck in the middle of an 'anxious episode.' If that sounds like something you need, please read on.

If you're experiencing overly anxious feelings right now, and it's something new, it may be scaring the living you-know-what out of you. For example: You're in the living room watching television, trying to relax. Maybe your husband or partner is in the other room, and if you've got kids, they're playing quietly. (I know...that sounds impossible. But, for the sake of this example, let's pretend). Dinner's in the oven, the house is pretty clean, laundry folded, and you're feeling okay— at the moment. Suddenly, out of nowhere, your heart starts racing, you feel a little short of breath, and you haven't a clue what it is or where it came from. Your eyes widen, your focus turns away from the television and is placed completely upon the unwanted, unexplained and scary feelings going on inside your body.

My God, you think. *I'm going die! What's happening to me?* You then become acutely aware of the pounding sensation in your chest, your ears, the throbbing pulse in your neck, etc. You feel anxious, all right. And who wouldn't?

Just about the exact scenario happened to me shortly after I miscarried. Having already suffered several overly anxious moments didn't help, because I still didn't know what the heck they were. Whenever they happened, I couldn't stop them from scaring me into a deeper frenzy of fear. Looking back, I see contributors to my anxious feelings: obviously, my miscarriage itself. I was still in the grieving process, and the toll that took upon my mind, body, and spirit was, as you know, almost incomprehensible. Secondly, although no doctor ever told me this, my hormones were a complete mess. Let's face it—I went from being a four and a half months pregnant, to not being pregnant at all. Women who carry their babies to full term, delivering healthy bundles of joy, often go through hormonal 'crazy' periods afterwards. I think the same applies to the woman who miscarries. It certainly applied to me.

So, there you are, on the couch, scared out of your mind because your body is doing its own thing and you seemingly have no control over it. Here's where I really want you to listen: You do have some control over it. I thought I didn't, and you may feel the same. That's because no one ever told you what was going on inside your body—that your racing heart didn't mean you were having a heart attack, etc. Because you probably never experienced these terrifying feelings before, why would you gather tools to help you understand and get through it?

I remember the day after I had my D & C (the doctor had to remove the baby). I was home with my husband (at the time) and a couple of friends. The scene I described above happened to me, less the kids playing quietly, and I flipped. I stood up, paced, felt detached from my body, and was convinced my heart couldn't possibly beat that fast without doing me in. My husband was at a complete loss, as I was, and thank God one of my dear friends had the wits about him to have me sit, and he began rubbing my feet.

That helped calm me to a degree, but it didn't do the trick. Why? Several reasons. My mind kept repeating terrible things. My internal dialogue was horrific. *I'm going to die! What's happening to me? I can't breathe! Why is my heart racing? What's wrong with me?* As I constantly repeated this negative self talk, it cranked the adrenaline to into high gear. The more afraid I got, the more adrenaline was created. A perfectly normal reaction to fear, but in the case of an anxiety attack, or anxious episode, where there's no imminent danger, a very self-destructive thing to do. I called my doctor, and you know what he said? "Get some sleeping pills and take half. There's nothing wrong. You're just upset."

Wow. I read the words and can't believe it. What a thing to say to someone going through that—especially from a doctor! (Not a knock to doctors. This one was a bit on the insensitive side). I didn't know what was wrong and like most people would, I followed the doctor's advice. If sleeping pills would get me off the crazy roller coaster ride I was on, I'd take one. At that point, I think I would have done anything to get rid of the nasty sensations ripping through my body. Off my husband went, shortly returning with some over-the-counter sleeping pills. I took half of one, and in about twenty minutes, was a complete zombie.

I need to interject something: You know I'm not a doctor—I advocate seeing one if you experience any unusual symptoms like the ones mentioned above, or anything else. I do not advocate taking sleeping pills to get you through an anxious moment. Believe me, I felt terrible as a result.

Let's move forward. What will *help*? If you've seen a doctor and know your symptoms are anxiety, what will get you through it? Counseling? Yes, that helps. If your doctor prescribed medication for what probably is a short period of time, it may help to a degree, but it won't give you the skills to get through an anxious moment. Even on medication, anxiety often rears its ugly head. I know because my doctor (years later) had me try several anti-anxiety medications. They usually made me feel worse, and I, under my doctor's supervision, stopped taking them. Finally, one worked and took the edge off, but didn't get rid of the attacks. That was up to me. My brain had to learn how to cope with anxious episodes, and a pill couldn't teach me that. Therapy helps, and what I'm going to share helps.

After you've seen a doctor and it's been determined you're suffering from anxious feelings: Don't convince yourself you're going to die by repeating that fearful thought over and over in your head like a record that's stuck. I used to do it all the time when I didn't know what the heck anxiety attacks were. Boy, did I make it worse by literally scaring myself into a longer-lasting, more severe anxiety attack. What does work is to gently remind yourself that although the feelings stink, because they do, they *will pass.* Your anxious moment won't last forever. (I know it feels like it will.) As a matter of fact, in about twenty-minutes, your body will calm down. It's amazing how our bodies know how to regulate themselves, but we can help them along during an anxious episode. It's critical you realize the scary sensations you're experiencing will go away—and believe it. It may take a while to train you brain into believing this because you're so scared. By repeating over and over again the positive message that your anxiety will not kill you and *will pass*, you're getting closer to convincing your brain it's the truth. The scary sensations brought on by anxiety will stick around longer if you reinforce them with negative messages, i.e., I am going to die or flip out. Instead, please try to use the positive ones, i.e., I'm going to be okay, this stinks but I'll get through it, I need to focus on my breathing and take air in nice and deep, etc. *What? Think positive when I'm scared out of my mind?* Yes. Just because it's normal to be afraid when you're having an anxious episode, doesn't mean you should magnify that fear. Your breath is shallow because you're scared, and that's the time you need to make yourself breathe deeply. When you think about it, it's a normal reaction to breathe shallowly when we're afraid, no matter what the reason. In your case, if you're feeling anxious and you can't figure out why, the only piece missing is the actual frightening event. Your body is reacting as if you were in a very frightening situation, and you gasp for air. At this point, taking deep breaths in through your nose and exhaling through your mouth needs to be done. Keep doing it. Take the scary thoughts racing through your head and do your best to replace them with the ones mentioned above, or some of your own. Whatever works for you. Just make sure it's positive. I'm not suggesting you deny your anxious feelings. That doesn't work, either. Going with them, admitting they're present, but negating their effects with positive messages is key to getting through your anxious feelings. I can't promise they'll go away completely, but I can promise these techniques will help. If they don't, and that's perfectly reasonable, please see your doctor for some help and begin working on controlling your anxiety and eventually, being able to put your anxious feelings out like a fire at its first spark.

Many times during an anxious moment, you feel dizzy, lightheaded, and possibly some tingly, numb feelings in your hands or around your mouth. This is because you're hyperventilating. When you breathe shallowly, (your chest rises up and down when you breathe instead of your stomach), your levels of carbon dioxide get all out of whack, and *that* makes you feel dizzy, etc. If you need to, (and this *works)*, grab a paper bag and breathe in and out of it until you begin to feel your body come back to normal. It will happen. The paper bag remedy is not an old-wives tale. Breathing in and out if it regulates your carbon dioxide level, bringing it back to normal. When this happens, the lightheadedness, etc., goes away. Sounds silly, but it works. Heck, I used to drive around with a paper bag under the seat of my car! Rarely did I need it, but it was there if I did. That alone provided me with a much needed sense of security.

Anxiety is something that can save our lives. It's only a bad thing when it's felt for the wrong reasons and often out of the blue. Anxiety, or increased levels of adrenaline, is what gives us the strength we need to get ourselves out of a bad situation. It's called the "Fight or Flight" response. If you're in the woods and bear starts to chase you, you're going to feel anxious! Thank, God for that. Your anxiety, or fear with a good reason, will give you the boost you need to run like there's no tomorrow, out of harm's way. All that adrenaline serves a purpose during a period of danger. However, that same adrenaline and reaction, (as if there's a bear chasing you in your living room), has no place to go, no purpose to serve, and that's why you end up suffering a horrible anxious moment. Your body's telling you there's something to be afraid of, reacting exactly as if there really were, and you end up feeling like you're about to flip. That's the lay-person's way of explaining your anxiety, and after all, that's what I am.

You know what your body dictates. If you feel dizzy and need to sit, breathe deeply, and let it pass, then that's what you need to do. I often did that, and on the flip side, I also felt the need to move around when I became anxious. There wasn't any rhyme or reason to it, no formula, etc. Sometimes my body told me to do something to burn off the extra adrenaline. Like what? I cleaned. I still clean a lot when I'm anxious. I suppose it's a productive use of the extra adrenaline, because I end up with spotless house! The feeling to get up and move didn't come, however, until I learned what my anxiety was and how to take control over the awful feelings it caused. I literally had to reprogram my brain so that it would believe the anxious moment would pass, and believe it or not, I am still working on that today. It's a constant process for me. With many of you, it's probably a temporary thing and you won't be like I am. I don't want to scare you into thinking just because you had an anxious moment, you're going to have them forever. Not true. The anxiety you're experiencing was brought on a traumatic event, your miscarriage. That's so painful you became overloaded and the anxiety crept in. With me, my miscarriage did make my anxiety worse, but anxiety also runs in my family. Heredity is a factor with me, and more than likely isn't with you. If you discover it is, take heart and know your life won't be spent in a perpetual state of anxiety. Give yourself a break right now and realize you're in the middle of a painful healing process and have suffered a great loss. If you feel lousy, there's a darn good reason for it and you will get through it.

Sometimes, anxiety made me feel like crying. (It still can.) When that happened, I did. Especially after my miscarriage. There were so many terrible emotions swimming around in my head. My body's way of releasing the pressure was to cry. When life gets to be too much, crying can be very cleansing. When I feel the need to cry, I allow it to happen, and afterwards, my chest is lighter and I feel like a load's been lifted off my shoulders. It isn't a permanent fix, but it helps me to move forward with a renewed sense of strength.

Tears aren't necessarily a bad thing. I used to think they were, but I believe tears make room for better feelings to come into our lives and hearts. Like a champagne bottle that's been shaken, there may times when you feel like you're going to pop. If you're at work and bursting into tears wouldn't cut it, promise to give yourself permission to cry later. It's okay, normal, and you deserve, even owe it to yourself, to let your feelings out.

Trust me when I say that if you don't allow yourself to feel, good and bad, you're making your anxious feelings worse, and inhibiting your growth and healing. I've walked both roads, and I am convinced that no good comes from allowing things to fester.

Breathe, think positively, try not to be afraid, cry if you need to, seek help if you need it, believe you'll be okay, the moment will pass— and never give up on yourself.

My Story, as published in: *Conquering Panic and Anxiety Disorders, Success Stories, Strategies and other Good News*, Jenna Glatzer, Editor, With Commentaries by Paul Foxman, PH.D.

Winning My Battle With Anxiety

I was very outgoing as a child. I'd put on plays in front of my parents, sing to records, and put on shows. I was like that all through both elementary school and high school. Nothing scared me, and my aspirations were high.

I began college as a Theater major and switched midstream to a Communications major. I pictured myself as the next big 'News Anchor.' I'd even auditioned at the Connecticut School of Broadcasting, impromptu, and got accepted.

At the age of twenty, during my sophomore year in college, I lost most of the sight in my left eye. To say I was frightened is an understatement. I was terrified. But, I handled it like a trooper, even on those nights when I was alone in the hospital not knowing what was wrong with me. When family visited, I appeared strong. At night, I cried alone.

Shortly after I got out of the hospital I went to see a stage production of *Fiddler on the Roof*. I remember it well because that was the first of many, many terrifying experiences. It was when I had my first anxiety attack.

During the show, my heart began racing so fast I thought I was dying. My chest constricted, and I couldn't get enough air. I hyperventilated. The more I panicked, the worse it got. I ran up the isle of the theater and headed straight for the phone. I needed to talk to my parents. I didn't know why, but their voices were what I needed to hear. I thought I was going crazy.

Immediately, my doctor was contacted to see if any of the medications I was given for my detached retina were the cause. The answer was no. I was told to go home and lay down.

61

The subject wasn't brought up again, but I suffered the attacks in agonizing silence.

About seven months after my loss of sght, I was out with my fiancé (at the time). Suddenly, I couldn't see with *both* eyes open. My heart began to race again as we rushed to the hospital. By the time we arrived, my verbal and motor skills were gone and the entire left side of my body was numb. You could have cut off my left arm and I wouldn't have felt it. I was screaming inside but when the nurse asked me to describe what I was feeling, all I could get out was, "Bah, ah." I couldn't form any words, (although I knew what I wanted to say), and I thought for certain that either I was having a stroke or was going to die of a brain tumor.

Well, fortunately, I was diagnosed with what's called a "classic migraine," which impairs verbal and motor skills. I regained those in about twenty minutes, and then I got the worst headache I'd ever had in my life. The doctor said it was stress-induced. It hasn't happened since, thank God.

And that was that.

As time went by my attacks came in cycles. They subsided for some time while in college, but shortly after I got married they seemed to come 'out of the blue.' Not often, but each time they were frightening. I didn't know then what I know now, and as I reflect back, I can see where I literally talked myself into a worse frenzy.

I didn't have the courage to seek any help. I thought this was something I just had to live with. I'd been examined by doctors for my eye and for the classic migraine and all of the test results said I was just fine.

So, I went on with my life.

At 25 I suffered a miscarriage. The baby didn't abort itself; it died in my womb and the doctors had to remove it. I was sixteen weeks pregnant at the time. When I got home from the hospital, I wanted to grieve, but my husband (at the time) and I were on different wavelengths. He thought I should get on with it and over it, and I just couldn't let go of my loss or my grief. That's when my anxiety attacks came back with a vengeance. I had heart palpitations that were so frightening I thought I'd have a heart attack. I worked for a ski area and commuted to New Hampshire, many times driving several hours alone, on weekends and suffered some horrific anxiety attacks while driving. He (my ex-husband) didn't really understand what was going on with me or sympathize very much. I can't blame him for not understanding it, but it didn't make it easier.

I kept it inside. And it festered.

At the age of twenty-seven my husband and I split up. My anxiety attacks grew worse and worse until it almost got to the point where I couldn't function. But, I forced myself to. I went to work, I drove even when my hands were so numb I couldn't feel them, and I talked to people when inside it took every ounce of strength I had to appear 'normal.'. It was exhausting. I was petrified. I couldn't eat alone for fear I'd choke. I couldn't eat in restaurants for fear of embarrassment. I'd stare at a plate of food and literally be starving—unable to get it down.

The advent of my divorce really was the catalyst to my first encounter with professional help. What originally was to be marriage counseling turned out to be individual talk therapy. I knew my marriage was over, but the anxiety needed to be dealt with, and this proved to be the beginning of my journey.

Adjusting after the divorce along with dealing with my anxiety attacks was quite challenging. It was very multilayered. I found that talk therapy helped. Not just with the divorce, but with the anxiety.

The talk therapy ended after about a year and a half when my therapist moved to another state. However, the knowledge and insight I gained was invaluable and put me on the path to recovery.

In the years that passed, I had my bouts with anxiety. I did extensive research on the subject and read countless self-help books. I was always reaching for more answers, for more assurance. As a result, I knew better how to deal with the attacks. The negative self-talk and the fear of loss of control diminished as I developed the ability to handle the attacks with my mind by gently talking my way through them.

They didn't completely go away, however.

In 1996 I met my fiancé. One of the biggest challenges he helped me to meet, unknowingly, was facing my anxiety. He is a pilot, and on one of our very first dates, he surprised me with a trip to the airport to take his plane for a flight. As my heart raced madly (for I'd never been on a smaller plane), I decided to face my fear. That flight was one of the most beautiful things I've ever experienced. Had I succumbed to my fear, I would never have seen the beautiful moon and stars on that clear and magical night. That taught me a wonderful lesson. I was stronger than my anxiety. I just needed to draw upon my strength.

In 1997 I went to a new primary doctor for severe intestinal pain. Upon examination, she told me that I had a stomach condition caused by Chronic Anxiety Disorder. She had only a brief idea of my history. But, after several questions, etc., she wisely came to her diagnosis. It was then that I began some more talk therapy, on her advise, and started taking a small amount of medicine, called Klonopin, to relieve some of the symptoms of anxiety.

In 1997 I became the lead singer of a wedding band. During my audition my anxiety got so bad that I could feel my knees knocking, and my lips were tingling! Try singing like that! But, somehow I made it through and got in. There was more than one "gig" where I'd feel my hands and mouth get tingly, and my legs would begin to buckle. But, I went on and made myself do it. I think that it pushed me further into discovering my own inner strength. If I could handle an anxiety attack in front of three hundred people (and believe me, it wasn't easy as I clung to the microphone stand to hold me up), then I could conquer this!

In the years that have passed, I have continued my research on anxiety. I still read many books dealing with the subject and put into practice many of the psychological things that help keep anxiety attacks at bay and/or under control.

I no longer use talk therapy, but what I learned in the process will stay with me forever.

It's not a battle that's won overnight, although the disorder seems to appear overnight. The road is long, and there are many ways to effectively treat anxiety. I think the most important things in helping a sufferer of anxiety are the support of those who love you, understanding the disorder, the faith that you will overcome it, and the knowledge that you are not alone in your struggle.

Believe me, you are not.

A big thank you to Anna for sharing her wonderful talent as a Reiki Master, and more importantly, for sharing her touching story of going through not one, but five miscarriages.

Anna's Story and What is Reiki?
Anna Pizzoferatto

Anna's Story

Miscarriage...just the word alone is able to stir within me twenty-year-old emotional debris. I will now go back in time and share with you my story. My first pregnancy ended abruptly New Year's Eve. I had barely completed my second month. For a girl who would pass out just being in a hospital, I would say the experience rates as traumatic. There I was, New Year's Eve under bright lights and surrounded by strangers, while my baby's remains cannot even be discerned or given a respectful goodbye. From that day on I had labeled New Year's as unlucky. I hated its approach.

My second pregnancy went to term. I just loved being pregnant and feeling this beautiful soul develop in my womb. I remember how real it all became when all the baby gifts from a shower flooded the house. I recall cheerfully saying to my husband "It looks like someone is moving in!" The delivery almost robbed me of my precious baby.

I was in heavy labor for 36 hours. I paced and paced while I meet shift after shift of medical staff. It finally took the nurse from "hell" who ended up saving my baby. She went wild when she realized just what was going on. I was in labor way too long to be good for my baby. She must have called for help. Thank God she took command. My quiet room became flooded with an army of medical personnel and bright lights. The nurse made me stop pacing and lie down. She insisted that I be induced. I imagine my doctor was somewhere in the mix. After some major pushing my son was born. He was quickly whisked away. I knew that the cleanup was taking way too long. I did not even get to hold him.

I was rolled off to my room and then gently told that my baby Nathan might not make it. Because of long labor without intervention, he had started breathing inside of me filling his tiny lungs were with fluid. I distinctly remember my reaction to the somber news. I looked at my husband and very calmly said, "I know he will make it." After nine days in intensive care, I finally got to bring my sweet baby home. I later learned his name means "Gift from God." I knew that I was truly blessed.

It did not take long for me to start dreaming of a second child. I came from a large Italian family and was determined to give Nathan a sibling. What happened after that was a blur of tears and fertility specialists. I had a second New Year's miscarriage followed by three more losses. I had become so accustomed to the routine that I drove myself to the doctor, had my D&C. and drove myself home. The pattern was the same. I got pregnant, felt all the right physical changes, and then to my horror would find myself feeling "normal" as I prepared for yet another sullen trip to the doctor's office.

The miscarriages were all devastating and without any apparent reason. The last one was the worst because it coincided with the birth of my nephew. It was the death of my dream. To this day my nephew's birthday party is a bit hard to take.

I can't say I coped well with all my losses. I tried real hard to be "strong" and keep on going. At that point in time Reiki had not yet entered my life so I just did the best I could. I repressed many more tears than what I had shed. Some of those tears have come up to be felt...twenty years later. It is no coincidence that I was asked to write this piece. It seems that the gentle hand of Reiki has provided me with this opportunity for mutual healing.

What is Reiki?

Anyone who has had the experience of losing a much wanted child knows that the pain cuts deep, long and hard. In my effort to have a family I had six pregnancies, five of which ended in miscarriage. The last loss was 15 years ago. The pain that I had to endure could have been easier to pass through had I known about Reiki.

Between the agony of the miscarriages and the hollowness of an unfulfilling marriage, I was called to Reiki years later. I am now Usui and Karuna(c) Reiki Master specializing in Reiki distance healing.

Reiki is a healing modality which has been used through the ages by the holiest of healers. Jesus and Buddha are just two of the more famous practitioners of this powerful healing art. When we hear of the miracles produced by historical healers and their students we never hear the term "Reiki" associated with the extraordinary events.

No need to worry about the name. It so happens that the method of tapping into this energy was rediscovered by a Japanese man, Dr. Usui, hence the Japanese name. One need not be concerned as to the label given this energy. The name is of no consequence. What is worthy of your attention is its benevolent source and healing power. The energy

Reiki practitioners direct toward recipients is of an intelligent and divine nature. The intelligence is privy to the precise type of healing needed, be it physical, spiritual or emotional. The area that requires the most urgent healing may indeed *not* be what the recipient had requested. One need only trust this divine intelligence.

There are several ways to receive a Reiki treatment. The Reiki practitioner can place their hands on the recipient allowing the energy to flow, or it can be received through projection of the energy by the Reiki practitioner. How one chooses to have a Reiki session does not influence the outcome. It is a matter of preference. You get what you need regardless of delivery.

Can Reiki help everyone? The only real limitation to its possibilities is the lack of desire for healing. If, on a soul level, an individual does not want the energy, it will not be accepted. Reiki cannot be forced on an individual. We have free will and have the right to choose not to heal.

There is tremendous potential in using Reiki to help parents process the events of the loss rather than turn the pain inward where it will eventually fester into disease. Reiki helps one pass through the pain in a gentle and safe fashion. Only by acknowledging and feeling the pain can one then hope to settle into a position of acceptance. Without acceptance, the inherent resistance intensifies the pain and breeds bitterness among other emotions which prevents one from joining the ranks of the living. Bitterness and envy do nothing to enhance the quality of life. The legacy of a child conceived in love should be reflected in a life that exudes joyous participation. Reiki gently helps you get to that place.

Reiki should not be used as a substitute for medical care. It should complement professional medical/psychological care.

Anna Pizzoferrato is a certified Reiki and Shamballa Master/Teacher. Her passion and specialty is Reiki Distance Energy Healing. Her website offers a free Reiki-charged sunset as well a monthly complimentary drawing. Learn more about Anna and Reiki on her website, ReikiWithTrust.com.

Relax—What's That?

Do you ever relax? Do you even remember what it feels like to be relaxed? I still battle with this, but fortunately have found ways to help myself relax. When your mind is constantly in overdrive, as it very well may be right now, it's tough to get your mind, body, and spirit aligned into a state of relaxation. When your thoughts are sad, negative, troubled…your physical self mimics your thoughts. So, you end up with trouble sleeping or tight, sore shoulders that don't seem to want to move down, away from your ears. I've been there, still experience it, but there are ways to help you settle down so you can at least enjoy some good, cleansing deep breaths and feel your body become less tense. Don't lose hope! I've also found that by removing myself from a place of negativity (let's say it's home because I'm feeling stressed and depressed), and just go out, even to the grocery store, it helps (and I can't stand grocery shopping). Changing your environment often leads to a state change. You step away from yourself a bit because you have to. When you're driving you've got to focus. At the market, you're around many people and that helps. Even though you may feel uptight, as you get your mind on other things, the tightness in your body starts to let go. It's easy to slip back, getting all wound up like a big knot. However, the simplest of things can help your mind and body learn to relax again. I've had to teach myself how to relax because over the years I let life's tougher times stay inside of me and I ended up constantly unable to relax. It wasn't until the end of the day, after I'd worn myself out from working, thinking, crying, cleaning, that I'd literally plop into the chair and nod off. But, is that really relaxation? I think it's more like exhaustion. I want to be awake and enjoy the feeling of relaxation throughout my mind and body. Perhaps you're like me and need a few tips on how to get there.

I'm one of those people who has a tough time relaxing, period. Compound that with a stressful or painful event, like my miscarriage, and forget it. I needed all the help I could get. I remember feeling like my insides and mind were constantly in fast forward, even when I was still. I couldn't stop thinking, and most of my thoughts were so sad. My sleep was affected (I didn't sleep enough), and I always felt exhausted. I didn't know how to relax anymore, and I craved it so much. Do you feel the same way?

If you have children, you may think you don't have the time to relax—or you might feel guilty relaxing. Because relaxing will take up a chunk of time you simply don't have, you may toss the idea of relaxing out the window and try to go on the way you are. Before I learned how to relax, I did the same thing. Believe me, it did me no good. I went for years without relaxing—or knowing what it was! Gone were the days when I relaxed without thinking about it, and I surmise that was and still remains a lot of my problem today. I *think* too much about relaxing, something which used to come so naturally— without any thought. That's what stress will do—what life itself often does. When you're on overload, it's as if your brain forgets the meaning of relaxation, and once again, we need to retrain our brains—teaching ourselves the meaning of relaxation and learning how to reach that state.

The stress of my miscarriage caused me to walk around most of the time in a perpetual state of being *wired and tired* simultaneously. I'm still like that, except for one very important difference: I take time to relax—even if only for a few moments, using effective techniques I've found, forcing my mind and body into a state of relaxation. Oh, and boy is my mind stubborn. It'll make me feel guilty for relaxing or unable to because there's so much to do around the house, or another book to work on, a poem, a website, whatever! There comes a time when I have to say: *Stop, sit, breathe, relax.* As far as the guilt associated with relaxing goes, I've tried to chuck it out the window, too. You may feel like you've *got* to clean the house, work on a report, do something with your children, wash the kitchen floor. While all those thing may need to be done, if you don't take the time to recharge your batteries, you'll end up feeling completely spent with little energy to do any of it, including healing from your miscarriage. You may also end up like I did—so worn down I literally ended up with a pneumonia the summer after my miscarriage. Please, don't let that happen to you. Take the time, even if you've only got five minutes, to refresh, rejuvenate—*relax*. As with most of what I've mentioned so far, I wish I knew then (when I miscarried) what I know now.

Some good news: You don't need to commit hours at a time to practice relaxation techniques. Whether you've got twenty-minutes or a few minutes, you can relax. If you're standing in line at the grocery store or waiting at a stop light—you can relax. Particularly now, with so much racing through your mind, you need to give yourself a break. So much of your energy is spent on worry, fear, sadness, and depression. Energy, just like gas in a car, runs out. Relaxation techniques fill your tank up so you can get through the rest of the day, and feel better doing it.

Perhaps you think watching television is relaxing. How many times have you heard, "Why don't you just sit down, watch TV and relax?" I heard it a lot and used to say it to others. However, if you think about it, does watching TV really make you *feel* relaxed? Maybe if you felt more 'normal' right now, it would. I can tell you this, when I was absorbed in grief and wound up tighter than a drum, watching television didn't relax me. My body didn't loosen up. My breathing didn't become deeper—less shallow. My neck didn't feel less stiff, and my headache didn't go away. I didn't feel less like crying, and I certainly didn't feel refreshed. I think the only thing television did for me was to *distract* me from my pain, temporarily. I'm not implying it's a bad thing, but in the long run, I wasn't teaching myself how to relax and my mind, body, and spirit. I wasn't getting any of the benefits *true* relaxation brings. As a matter of fact, the moment I got up to resume 'real life,' I felt just as wound up as I did prior to turning on the television.

As I said, I didn't know about the relaxation techniques I'm going to share with you after I miscarried, but I clearly see how I would have been so much better off had I known about them. Miscarriage fallout just doesn't go away, and when I learned how to relax, it helped me, even years later, to release much of the pain I still carried with me. Relaxation has proved invaluable in managing my anxiety. Sharing some techniques with you, as you face what may seem an insurmountable obstacle of sadness, is so important to me. My wish is for you to find at least one relaxation technique that feels right to you. Just as we're all individuals, we have different ways of relaxing. Pick and choose. Try one, and if it doesn't do the trick, don't despair. Just move onto another. If nothing seems to work, you may need a bit of professional help to put you on the right path. Please don't be afraid. I sought help, and know with everything I am that it takes more courage to seek help than to remain in a state you no longer wish to be in. Please don't allow your uncomfortable state to become your comfort zone. You *deserve* to feel better. You're entitled to learn how to relax and to give that gift to yourself. Relaxation helps in your overall healing process, and smoothes out some of the bumps in the road you're on.

So, what makes me an expert in relaxation techniques? I'm not. I'm simply a woman who learned through a lot of trial and error some ways to help calm my mind and body.

If you're afraid you haven't a moment to spare, I think you'll be pleasantly surprised at how quickly you can relax, giving your spirit a chance to open up.

I must interject something here: Shortly after my miscarriage, my emotions were so volatile that when I did try to relax, I often ended up crying. I can't speak as a medical expert, but I let the tears come. In my opinion, they needed to get out, and by slowing myself down and doing what I often avoided (thinking), I allowed my body to release pent up tears. I experienced a sort of inner cleansing, if you will, and it happened far more than once. It still happens today when I'm going through a particularly difficult time. I say this so you'll be aware that you're not alone if this happens to you. We don't create these feelings, they simply exist. That doesn't take away from their very real presence in our lives, or diminish their meaning in any way. Actually, it's quite the opposite. By allowing ourselves to feel, we acknowledge our feelings.

If you don't have ten to twenty minutes to dedicate towards relaxing, let me give you a few pointers that will work wonders in a matter of seconds—after you get the hang of it. Anything new takes practice.

Let's say you're on your way home from work. It was a busy day, so you weren't allowed the time to think about the pain you're in after miscarriage. In the back of your mind, it lingered—and you felt it. But, work proved to be a great escape route, and you dove into your job with vigor.

However, now you're alone in your car. Whenever I was alone in my car, I wanted to cry. It was time for me with no one to distract me, interrupt me, or simply be around me. I was free to feel whatever I wanted and just let it come out. That's not a bad thing, but breaking down while behind the wheel isn't safe for you or others on the road. I realize that sometimes you can't help it, but if you find you're really sobbing out of control, please pull over like I sometimes had to do.

Okay, so whether or not you've had a cry in your car, you're now on your way to the grocery store. While walking up and down the isles, you find yourself feeling more and more uptight. Perhaps your breathing is growing shallow, and you're starting to get light-headed. I felt this way more times than I can count. As you make your way through the store, you find yourself in the baby food isle and want to scream. You make it through, but by the time you get in line to check out your food, you feel like you're going to flip.

Talk about tense. There you are surrounded by people, having just gone through a very tragic event, and each second feels like an eternity between you and finally reaching the safe haven of your car. What to do?

Focus on your breathing. Right then and there, do it. No one will know what you're doing, because there's nothing to see. Breathe in through your nose for a count of two, and out through your mouth for a count of four. Nobody will stare at you, because you're counting to yourself. In through the nose for a count of two, out through your mouth for a count of four. When you count, don't do it quickly. Try to keep it even and fairly slow. Count one-one thousand, two-one thousand, etc. By the time you have to place your food on the belt, you'll feel calmer and more pulled together. Why? You've taken your mind off of freaking out, or wanting to, and placed it on one thing alone—your breathing. By doing this, you've not only regulated your breathing and given your body the oxygen it needs (you were probably hyperventilating prior to doing this exercise), you've also relaxed your chest muscles and all the other muscles in your body. If this works for you, do it whenever you feel tense, anxious, and in need of relaxation. It's a very quick fix to a sometimes debilitating problem. It doesn't mean you won't feel stressed later, or need to cry to release your emotions, but it'll get you through a tough spot, fast.

Note: Deep breathing is the foundation of many other relaxation exercises.

After doing this repeatedly, it can become a part of your life. When I'm at home or in my car, and feel myself getting wound up, I do this exercise. It helped when I first started focusing on my breathing, and still does.

This simple exercise can be taken a step further. Progressive Muscle Relaxation— It involves tensing, then relaxing the body muscles from head to toe. (I've heard that this can increase blood pressure temporarily, so check with your doctor, first.)

Wear loose, comfortable clothing and find a spot to sit or lie down that's also comfortable. It can be the floor, your bed, an exercise mat— whatever suits you. I always begin this relaxation technique by focusing on my breathing for about a minute or so. This helps slow down my often racing mind and starts relaxing my tense body.

Start with the muscles in your face and frown hard for a count of five, counting fairly slowly, then relax all your muscles. You'll be amazed at how relaxed your face alone feels after you do this. Do the same for the other muscles in your face, holding for the same count of five, and then releasing: your jaw (clenching it), tightly closing your eyes, raising your eyebrows. Feel the tension in these muscles, and then release.

Now it's time to move on to other muscle groups, repeating the same exercise for a count of five, then releasing: raise your shoulders, tighten your arms, your chest, your back, legs, etc.—until you've tensed and relaxed your whole body, from your face all the way down to your feet. I liken this exercise to getting a massage without leaving the house. I carry a lot of tension in my body, and if you're anything like me, you'll benefit greatly from this short and easy relaxation technique.

Often, deep breathing is incorporated into guided meditation tapes. I find them to be very helpful. A guided meditation tape (there are hundreds) typically has some very soothing background music playing, while someone speaks in a very calm, even tone. One of my favorites begins with the breathing technique I mentioned above and then goes on to relax the entire body, beginning with the feet and working your way up to the head. (The same as the Progressive Muscle Relaxation exercise, only you begin with your feet.) After that, the tape guides you on a journey into an extremely vivid, beautiful, peaceful forest. The guided meditation concludes with 'me' picturing, or visualizing, how I want to be in the present moment. I always see myself smiling, full of confidence, strong and healthy. I'm happy when I see myself as I wish to be and know deep inside that it's possible.

When I'm done with this guided meditation tape, I'm always amazed at how different I feel. My entire body is relaxed. My shoulders, which I tend to carry up somewhere around my ears, are down where they're supposed to be. My breathing is naturally calmer and easier— my chest area more open.

This feeling, however, doesn't last forever. I'm not trying to take away from it's importance, but I am stressing this for a reason. Life is life, and you aren't living it through a guided meditation tape 24/7. But you *always* have the tape, and what it teaches you, to fall back on. Eventually, your mind will be able to take you to that beautiful, peaceful state upon recall, whenever you need it—even standing in line at a grocery store. The key is listening to whatever tape you like enough, so that your brain holds onto that state of calm, storing it away for future reference. I think of my brain like a library. Whenever I need that book on calm, (or what the tape taught me), I go get it. The only way a book is added to my library is by repeating the guided meditation tape (or other techniques) until I can actually make my body feel the same relaxed sensation, simply by thinking about it. This proves very helpful if you're at work, or anywhere, and don't have the time nor the benefit of listening to a tape, but need to unwind in a hurry.

If guided meditation isn't for you, take heart. There are other things you can listen to that have natural calming effects on the mind and body. Music, for one. I'm not talking about cranking Springstein, (nothing against Bruce—I like his music). If you have any New Age tapes or CDs with soothing music and no heavy orchestration or loud notes, they'll do the trick. Some examples would be: Enya, Yanni, Vengelis, etc. Just ask for help finding them in your local music store. Not only will you relax, you'll reap the benefits of some great music. There are some new tapes out under the name of Brain Sync, which are specifically designed to put you in what they call a 'theta state'—or very relaxed state, through music. I've yet to try them, but you can be sure they're on my list of things to do.

Don't forget, you can play relaxing music while in your car, cleaning the house, cooking...whatever. I don't advocate playing a guided meditation tape in your car (it doesn't work AND it's not safe), but music is different. It has the power to soothe you safely, wherever you are.

If you don't believe in the soothing power of music, think about this: How often have you felt edgy or irritated when music you hate is playing—especially loudly? If music has the power to make you feel wound up, it also has the power to make you feel calm.

Sing! You don't have to be a singer to sing. But, singing is calming if you can get yourself into it. You may find at the beginning of your healing process, it's tough to do. If that's the case, don't do it. However, if at some point you feel it's right, just do it. Singing elevates us, releases tension, and (another great bonus) forces us to breathe deeply, from the diaphragm. Sometimes, if you're not used to singing, you may feel dizzy. Just stop for a minute. There are so many benefits to singing. In a way, it's a form of meditation because you're focusing on the words, music, etc., giving your mind the detour it needs. Secondly, the pure calming effect of breathing properly is achieved when you sing. If you don't breathe from your belly when you belt out a tune, you're in for some very strained vocal cords. (Believe me, I know this. I sang with a band for about three years, and if I didn't breathe properly, I sounded like I had a frog stuck in my throat by the end of the night.) So, if you find your throat telling you to back off, remember to breathe from deep within and don't force your singing. Sing softly, if you want to. Remember, this is for your benefit, and even if you believe you 'can't sing'—it doesn't matter. You may not be the next great sensation, but that's not the point. The point is to do it if it feels right and good, regardless of how you sound, and rid yourself of some tension. Heck, I even bought myself a karaoke machine! It's like a little stress relieving 'toy' I turn to, and I can bring it along to the next summer BBQ for others to have fun with.

Side Note: Just the other day I was feeling like a bottle about to burst. What did I do? I went downstairs, turned on my karaoke machine, and started singing and dancing. To the average person strolling past the window, I might have looked like a nut! (No one walks past that window.) Even if someone did, would I care? *No.* Why? Because I'm beyond that point. If I want to sing, dance, and bring myself to a better place, that's my right (unless, of course, I'm keeping the neighbors up). Before I knew it, about an hour or so had past *and* the tears I'd felt coming on were gone. My body felt more relaxed, my breathing was deeper, my headache was gone, etc. It helped set the tone (pardon the pun) for the rest of the night. Had I not done this exercise in giving my mind a break and 'switching channels' if you will, I know how the evening would have turned out. I would have ended up crying and more than likely would have remained in a down mood until I went to bed.

Let's recap. So far, we've got deep breathing, Progressive Muscle Relaxation, guided meditation, soothing music, and singing in our toolbox of relaxation techniques. Now, onto yoga.

Yoga—The All Natural Stress Reliever

I have an terrific series of yoga tapes for the beginner that I love. They bring me to a place I can't seem to reach without them. Yoga forces me to stop my racing emotions, body, you name it, and do nothing but yoga. When I can't get a deep breath in, yoga opens my chest. When my muscles hurt from walking around like a huge knot of tangled yarn all day, yoga soothes, stretches, and relaxes my muscles. When my mind is on overload and I can't tell whether I'm sad, fearful, or feel like I'm 'losing it', yoga erases those feelings, centers me, and makes me realize that I'm okay. When my spirit needs attention, but I'm too preoccupied with my thoughts, yoga places me into a realm of calm and quiet. In that realm, I am better able to pray, listen to God, or simply feel the calming hand of our Creator touching me. An amazing feeling of connection to the universe takes place—even if only for ten or twenty minutes. There are so many wonderful things yoga does for me—I can't put it all into words. That'd be another book! Just know this: If you feel like flipping out too often, don't know which end is up, find yourself anxious, troubled, weeping all the time, snapping at those you love, and just plain tired from being so wound up all the time, yoga is worth a try. You've got nothing to lose and everything, including increased energy and flexibility, to gain. If it's okay with your doctor, do yourself a favor and try yoga. If you love it, you'll know it. If you don't, then it's simply not for you right now.

When going through any traumatic event, in this case, the terrible loss you've just experienced, you've probably noticed the buildup of stress. Compounded with the every day fast-paced, demanding life you already lead, you may be looking for simple ways to calm your nerves. Yoga, an ancient practice, offers time-tested ways to effectively and efficiently reduce stress in your life.

What does yoga do? Other than firm, tone, and make your body more flexible, it also soothes your nerves and calms your mind. Talk about getting two great benefits in one. You can get in shape while relaxing? You bet. Physically, emotionally, and spiritually.

Yoga's been used for centuries for both health and meditation purposes. Finally, doctors are seeing the link between nervous disorders (in my case anxiety disorder), stress (often a precursor for anxiety attacks), and disease—my own doctor is a perfect example of Western medicine meeting Eastern health practices. She's asked me about exercise, meditation, etc., suggesting I incorporate it into my daily life to help alleviate my anxiety. I've also learned through a sixteen-week anxiety program that *any* kind of exercise, mediation, yoga, etc., is essential to balancing the mind and body—keeping you healthy. This message has been reinforced through so many channels I can't help but believe in it. The benefits of yoga are supported not only by scientific research, showing that deep relaxation oxygenates the body and helps combat many diseases, but by my own personal experience with yoga. In addition, the deep oxygenation of the body ties in *so* closely with the deep breathing exercises I do—which are not yoga related.

I'm seeing some very common threads between the benefits of any relaxation technique on the mind, body, and spirit. Breathing is one of them.

More than likely, you feel the stress taking its toll on you. Even though stress is first experienced in your mind (where everything originates), you may find yourself dealing with symptoms which have manifested in your body. Like what? Headaches, tight, achy muscles, stomach disorders (a big one with me), shallow breathing, anxiety or panic, bouts of crying to relieve the built up tension, and more. Perhaps you're not sleeping well or not sleeping enough (my experience). When you're constantly feeling stressed and don't know how to lessen or rid yourself of it, it can lead to more serious conditions. I don't want that for you, for me—so if yoga, in all its beautiful, ancient simplicity, can help you without you having to take a pill, please give it a go when you're ready. I don't want your stress to be hanging around for so long that you end up at your doctor's office (like I did), complaining of very real symptoms which could have been avoided if you knew what I know now. (Boy, do I wish I knew it then!) After my miscarriage, my stress levels were so high, along with my constant anxiety attacks, I ended up on a prescription for my constantly upset and painful digestive tract. Now, years later, there's a name for what I have—IBS, or Irritable Bowel Syndrome. I often wonder if this could have been avoided had I practiced the techniques I do now—back then. My guts scream that it's true, so please take heart in what I'm sharing with you so you don't end up like I did. I allowed my emotions and stress to control me for so long my poor body just couldn't fight back anymore, and I ended up with some conditions that I know could have been avoided.

Yoga isn't something to be afraid of because you think you can't do it. I'm no yoga master, but the mere act of attempting the various postures, etc., is rejuvenating, requires focus, and is a fantastic reliever of tension and stress.

Yoga is a wonderful stress reducing technique!

I first started my yoga with a book explaining and illustrating different postures (I still refer to it) and stretching exercises to do after my yoga routine. So, how do I feel after a yoga session? My chest feels open, muscles loose and free, tension from my body and mind gone. However, because I often let my negative thinking take the wheel, the restfulness and peace I feel after yoga is washed away the moment I allow stress to take control. But, that's my motivation to keep practicing yoga and other relaxation techniques and exercises. Over time, my mind and body *have* learned to manage stress better, but it's an ongoing process. I will arrive, someday, at a place where I don't allow stress to control me—I'll control how I react to it and be a much healthier person as a result.

Yoga provides immediate stress relief. Wouldn't it be great if one yoga session was all it took? However, we know that's not the case. Try to think of yoga as a prescription for your stress. Your doctor probably wouldn't give you one pill and say, "Okay, that'll do it. Your stress will be under control forever." You'd refill your prescription and continue with it until it's time to stop. The same principle applies to yoga, less the drugs. What a wonderful thing! (You may or may not need a prescription, depending upon your level of stress, your symptoms, etc. See your doctor if you're feeling really lousy and also ask him/her about yoga before you begin. That applies to all the exercises I mention.)

I alternate yoga with other exercise routines to break things up a bit, but wanted to include it in this section of the book because it's such a fantastic way to put yourself in a brighter, lighter, more peaceful place—just what you may be craving right now.

Let's say I'm not the most coordinated person in the world, so certain postures are tough for me. If you're the same, don't worry. It's not how great you become at yoga (unless that's a personal goal). It's doing it that counts. In addition to my yoga book, I use a yoga ball with an instructional video and love it. (Rolling off the ball wasn't too fun—so be careful.)

The most amazing thing about yoga is how much concentration it takes—without even realizing it. I believe that's one of the keys to stress reduction of any kind. When you attempt a yoga posture, you have no choice but to focus on what you're doing. The act of focusing works like a guided meditation or deep breathing exercise. Your mind is taken away from your problems, fears, worries, and sadness, providing the respite you need.

When practicing yoga, your mind is taken off yourself, your pain, off of everything—except for what you're doing at that moment. You are forced into living in the now *and enjoying it.*

Yoga helps your entire being— mind, body, and spirit. That's tough combination to beat, and better yet, it doesn't require a lot of time or money. Just a little patience.

I highly recommend getting yourself a beginner's guide to yoga book or a beginner's video tape—if yoga sounds like it's for you.

Tai Chi follows suit with yoga and can make a huge difference in how you feel. Much like yoga, Tai Chi is highly recommended for stress reduction and more— strengthening, flexibility, and toning to name a few. Here are some examples of medical conditions Tai Chi can help with: anxiety, breathing trouble, fatigue, depression, and muscle tension. Tai Chi incorporates deep breathing, relaxation, and gentle exercise. I use a Tai Chi video tape and follow as best I can. (The movements are slow—very flowing. They appear easier to do than they are, and it takes time to build the fluidity of those on the tape. Cut yourself some slack and don't get disheartened when you begin. Like anything, it takes practice— but the act of practicing is the fundamental key in obtaining yoga or Tai Chi 's benefits.)

Again, being somewhat of a 'klutz'—I recognize my accomplishments each time I manage to perform Tai Chi without losing my balance, etc. Remember to give yourself a pat on the back if you decide to try any of the relaxation techniques I've mentioned. Why? Because I know how difficult it is just to get motivated. When you do, you've conquered a huge mountain, and believe me, you deserve that pat.

In practicing Tai Chi, I get in touch with my core, my inner-self or spirit. When that happens, I'm reminded of who I am, how beautiful life can be, and how great it feels to finally relax. What a great feeling to breathe deeply without having to think about it!

The Importance of Exercise
in Relieving Tension

Just the word exercise used to scare me! I'd think, "I can't do that; it's too hard. I can't work out; I'm too out of shape." Well, guess what? Exercise doesn't need to be tough, painful or threatening, and it literally blasts the tension from your body and mind. There are forms of exercise that provide so many benefits yet are not threatening or out of reach. Can you walk? Try walking in place to a tape program in the comfort of your own home. If the weather's good, head outside if you want. Can you breathe? Try some fabulous breathing and resistance exercises in the comfort of your own space and watch the tension leave your body, and some inches and pounds, too. Do you clean your house? Realize that cleaning burns calories, focuses your mind on things other than your miscarriage, and leaves you with a sense of accomplishment. Is that treadmill still being used as a coat-rack? Give it a try, even if only for a few minutes while you watch your favorite show or, if you've got children, while they're sleeping or at school. You'd be amazed at what just ten minutes will do for you. Try three ten-minute increments of exercise per day, or every three days. It all adds up to thirty minutes of exercise per day—which is just what the doctor ordered! Break it up, break it down, and make exercise something that you can easily fit into your life. You don't have to spend a fortune on a gym membership—but, if you're more comfortable exercising around people, a gym membership is perfect for you. You'll also gain the benefit of some coaching by trained professionals. Not only will you feel motivated by those around you, you'll probably avoid injury because someone's there instructing you on how to exercise properly. It's all up to you. Whatever works—home, a gym, your street for a walk, the mall for a walk, a treadmill, some form of exercise to a tape, or creating your own program based around your schedule and activities. If you've got stairs in your house, just going up and down them a few times a day to start— is a great start. Please don't equate exercise with a monumental task you either can't do or don't have time for, and…always check with your doctor before you begin any exercise program.

I made a vow in 2004, 2005, and now into 2006 to exercise more. I did this for a couple of reasons: the obvious one of shaping up, and the other, which holds even greater importance—managing my stress. Stress makes you unhealthy, so what good would getting in better shape do if I weren't managing my stress, too? But, here's the key: *exercise is a natural stress reducer.* You can't help but manage your stress when you exercise, because your body won't have it any other way. When you exercise your body releases endorphins, and those are what give you the emotional lift. Although temporary, that emotional lift significantly reduces your stress level. Ever heard of the 'runner's high'? The endorphins are what causes that very real, uplifting feeling. I've come to the conclusion that I can't exercise without lowering my stress level. It's up to me to work out what's causing it, and in your case, it's very normal to feel stress as a byproduct of your miscarriage. I am sorry you have to experience those feelings, but I can offer some hope: *Although it's rough and you don't want to live it, things will get better over time and exercise can help relieve some of your tension as you move towards healing.*

I wish I started exercising a long time ago. Looking back, I know exercise would have done so much for me after my miscarriage. But, that's the funny thing about hindsight. However, when I do think about that terrible time in my life, I naturally turned towards one thing in particular I can remotely equate to exercise: I cleaned the house to the point of distraction. Back then, I didn't realize the physical activity was doing me good. I only knew I needed to do *something* other than think. It was driving me mad and pushing me further into a pit of depression. Cleaning the house gave my body something to do with all the adrenaline that was pumping through me as a result of being anxious all the time. I was like a rubber band ready to snap. Had I known more about exercise and the stress relieving techniques I mentioned, I would have done much more than clean the house incessantly. Because my mind was on such overload, I needed the suggestion to come from somebody. If someone asked, "Ellen, why don't you try a little exercise to help make you feel better?" I probably would have done it. I would have had reservations, thinking I was too out of shape or 'bummed out' to do it. But, eventually, I know I would have tried it because later on in life, after another traumatic event (my divorce), I did begin exercising. I remember it like yesterday: a step aerobic program I did at home. I don't want to stray from the subject, but divorce is another great loss and it's ranked right up there in the top ten most stressful life events. By that point I'd done enough reading to know the benefits of exercise went far beyond the physical. It didn't take my pain away, but it helped get me through it and controlled my overly-sensitized self. The same applies after a miscarriage: You're nerves are overly-sensitized, you're wound up like a knot, and at times you may fear you're going to explode. If that sounds like you, exercise is a tool that helps get those feelings under control. It won't make them go away and will not stop you from grieving. What it will do is make the road you're on a bit less bumpy because you'll feel stronger, therefore better able to cope.

Motivation. Boy, is it tough to get motivated. Even if life is going along just fine, exercise can be tough to begin. It was so difficult to 'just do it'—and that applies to many times in my life. I'd stick with it for a while and then allow myself to stop. Each time I let that happen, I found it just as difficult to get motivated again. It seems I've found the right combination of exercise programs this time around, and I'm pretty good at sticking to it. But, *the act of starting* was the toughest. I completely sympathize with anyone who's having a difficult time getting going. Know this: Once you do, and you give it a week (perhaps not every day of the week), you'll feel like you've achieved something. You have. Each time, never mind each week, I exercise, I feel better about myself. Not because I'm exercising, although that's part of it. But, doing something good for myself makes me feel better about myself. Allowing myself the time to be healthier is like giving myself a gift, and I, you, everyone deserves and is entitled to that gift. You've only got one you, and you are worth the time.

The benefits of exercising are more of a bonus—i.e., better health, lower cholesterol, losing a few pounds, toning up, *relieving stress.*

By not allowing my fears to keep me from exercising, I'm reaping the rewards.

Time: Exercise doesn't have to take a large chunk out of your day, can be done a thousand different ways, is something you can share with your children, should be tailored to your specific needs and physical health, and doesn't have to make you break out into a sweat, gasping for air. With some of my programs I may get a little winded, and that's normal because my body is demanding more oxygen as my heart rate increases (aerobic), but some of my exercise programs are entirely different—like Tai Chi, yoga, simple stretching exercises. (If you decide to start any exercise program, please check with your doctor first.)

If you've just miscarried, it may be too soon for you to begin exercising. When I miscarried, I spent the first week in tears practically all the time. But, it's what I needed. I see it was part of my healing process, and I had every right to grieve. Oh, how I wish someone told me that! So, the exercises I'm going to share with you are meant to be done when you're ready, and only if you feel exercise is right for you.

There's no right or wrong—but in the long run, you will do nothing but benefit from exercise whether you start in a week, a month, or a year. Exercise is important for all of us, and I'm sure I'm not the first person you've heard that from. Also, the exercises programs I use are very non-threatening, can be done if you're a beginner (I still consider myself to be one), and don't take up a large amount of time. They are meant to be gentle suggestions and certainly aren't the only ways of doing it. Also, exercise does not have to mean riding a stationary bike, working out to a video, or joining a gym. Exercise comes in many forms, and what you may not think of as exercise, actually is.

Here's a good example: I was talking to my mother on the phone, and she brought about an interesting point. If you decide you'd like to take a walk, that certainly counts as exercise and you can make it so much more than a walk. Bring a camera along, notice your surroundings, and take some photographs. Actually take the time to stop and smell those roses. Your body will love the fresh air and exercise, and your spirit will feel refreshed. It's amazing how many beautiful things in every day life go unnoticed. Just the other morning I was sitting at the kitchen table just after the sun came up. Looking out the window, I couldn't help but notice the brilliant azaleas that seemed to bloom overnight. Their petals were kissed by morning dew, and I became grateful for the beauty nature offers. I think I'll take my mother's advice, bring the dog along, and walk, observe, take notice, and appreciate what this wonderful earth has to give. Now that spring is here, it'll be wonderful, but even in the winter, there's beauty all around. Keep that in mind if you decide to take a walk. You may even get some amazing photographs, if you're a shutter-bug. Your walk can be a spiritually rewarding and emotionally cleansing experience.

I don't have children, but my sisters do, as do many of my friends. When I babysit, I realize how little time there is to do anything for yourself. If one child is sleeping, the other is often awake. If your child is sleeping, you may use that time to catch up on laundry, do a little cleaning, or take a break. Although I can't speak from experience because I don't have a child, I honestly realize that time is a very precious commodity for those of you who do have children. If you also work outside the home, it's even more precious. I bring this up because I want you to know that many of the exercises I suggest don't have to take much of your time. Recently, I read an article which said that a couple of ten minute workouts a day are better for you and result in superior results than let's say, one half-hour work out. There were a few reasons mentioned: People tend to stick with something that doesn't take much time, and you're boosting your body's metabolism, etc., twice a day instead of once. This results in more weight loss, if that's a goal for you, and in general, more people continue with exercising. Sounds like good news to me. I'm no expert—just read it in a magazine. But, it was written by an expert after an extensive study was performed on two groups of women. There may be a lot of fitness experts out there who disagree with what I've said, but please keep in mind that like most of us, I'm no expert, and I learned it from an article on fitness. I'll have to see for myself if it's true for me. My point: If you're pressed for time because of kids, a demanding job, or both, you don't need to fear beginning an exercise program for lack of time. We all can find ten or twenty minutes somewhere in our day—and that's all it takes. If you think about it, any amount of exercise is better than none, period.

Here's an example of making exercise fun if you're at home with a child and are strapped for time: My sister recently had her second baby. She also works out of the home. Needless to say, she's a busy woman! However, after her son was born, she felt like she had to exercise to get back into shape. The time to do it? She got creative.

After discovering she loved doing Pilates at home with a videotape as her guide, she began the work-out. My niece, who is almost three, is usually awake when my sister does her routine. So, what did she do? She got a little 'exercise mat' for her daughter, and when my sister does her Pilates for twenty minutes, my niece does her own little workout on her mat. This accomplishes three things: My sister gets to do her Pilates, my niece feels like she's doing something fun with Mommy, and because my niece is participating with my sister, she is occupied and doesn't need to be watched. She's already there! In the meantime, my nephew's usually having a grand time in his little seat that does about a thousand different things.

Also, when my sister takes the kids for a walk, she considers it more a 'power walk' than anything, which it is. There are two kids in that carriage, and the resistance alone makes the walk more of a work out. So, if you don't consider taking your child for a walk exercise, please reconsider! It's said that one of the most highly recommended forms of exercise is a one-mile aerobic walk. Well, put one or two kids in a carriage and get those legs moving, and that's exactly what you've got.

Remember, if you're like me and have no children, a walk is a walk. Whether you go alone, with your partner, or your dog, walking is great exercise, gets you out into the fresh air, and does wonders for relieving stress and anxiety. I can't help but think of an advertisement I once saw in a magazine. There was a picture of a dog with big, brown eyes, holding a leash in his mouth. Underneath the image it read: Think of him as a treadmill with fur.

Here's another example of how to incorporate your children into your exercise routine, and it doesn't even feel like exercise! I was talking to my best friend on the phone recently, and she said her husband was just getting in from taking a nature walk with her son. Wow, I thought. How wonderful! What a great way to include your child, or children, in your exercise routine. It seems so obvious, but we don't often think of something like a nature walk as exercise. It is! You're out there in the air, traversing paths and rocks, making those legs work and your heart pump. So, if there's not a moment to spare, and no one's around to watch the kids, take them out with you, or do what my sister does (with the exercise mat for her daughter), and make your child a part of your routine. I see women in my neighborhood all the time walking their babies, and no longer see it as simply 'taking the baby for a walk.' It's so much more. Mother's getting exercise, baby's getting fresh air, it's a change from being in the house, and a great stress reducer.

In terms of time and money, I used to think maintaining an exercise program would take large amounts of both. You know what? It's not true. I could have joined a gym. Heck, my sister is the manager of one! But, exercising at home is more comfortable for me, and there's no membership fee. I advocate gyms to anyone who likes and possibly needs the support of others to stick with a program. However, if you're like me, you can enjoy exercise at home, and the great benefits you'll derive from it will be your motivation. I tell you this from experience.

What do I do? While on the subject of walking, that's become one of my favorite at-home ways of exercising. It's so easy, boosts my metabolism, releases those endorphins, and I don't need to move any furniture around to do it. It's walking in place, and you get the same benefits (less the fresh air), as you do when walking outdoors. This is especially fantastic when the weather is lousy. I use a tape as my guide, and in as little as thirty minutes (including the stretching afterwards), I've completed a full, heart-healthy, one-mile aerobic walk that gives me the extra 'pep' I need to get through the day, and it helps my waistline, legs, butt, and the rest of me firm up. When I'm feeling more motivated, I do the longer version, burning more calories, working a bit harder, and feeling more accomplished when I'm finished. The point is, whether I do the short routine, or the longer one, I always end up with a feelings of satisfaction and stress relief when I'm done. Sometimes, I begin my routine with my head swimming with emotions. I may be depressed, worried, or overly concerned about something. Not long into my routine, my mind automatically is taken *away* from my worries, etc., and I'm in another place—a better one. That alone stops the stress dead it its tracks.

What else do I do at home? Well, deep breathing exercises are fabulous for relieving tension, filling your body with much needed oxygen, with the added benefit of losing inches and pounds. I do a program that combines deep breathing (that serves to oxygenate my body and relieve tension) with different, specific body positions. This program has a series of positions which target different parts of your body (even your face and neck), and the entire routine takes less than twenty minutes! It's also considered aerobic because you're increasing the level of oxygen in your body (by definition, that's aerobic). As a result, I give my metabolism a boost, burn fat, and I have the tape measure to prove I've lost inches. Not only is this routine fun and relatively easy to do, I always feel energized when I'm done. It's hard to feel depressed when you feel energized and refreshed. That applies to *all* forms of exercise.

Exercise gives your mind the break it needs and channels the negative emotions into something positive, leaving you stronger and better able to cope.

Recently, my VCR broke, and I wondered what to do in place of my exercise programs on tape. I could take the dog for a walk, for one, which I did. However, I'm one of those people who's referred to as a 'spaz' because I operate off of a lot of nervous energy. Without giving it much thought, I got creative. Also being a compulsive cleaner, I grabbed my duster and began to walk in place while I dusted. I thought it was going pretty well, and I was killing two birds with one stone. So, after I'd finished dusting, with my feet still walking in place, I reached for the dry-mop and went over the floors. Before I knew it, *more* than twenty minutes had passed and I wasn't done! The longer I cleaned, the more I increased the pace of my steps, just like on the video. To keep it safe, I then began to slow my pace as I wound down, bringing my heart rate back to normal. By the time I'd finished walking, cleaning, and stretching afterwards, I'd been working out for forty-five minutes and had an entirely dusted first floor! So, if you work out using tapes or DVDs and your player breaks, use your imagination and create your own exercise program.

Added Bonus: I actually saved time by incorporating the two.

It may sound strange, and you can't mix cleaning with every exercise program, but I want to share this because you may think you should be cleaning, not exercising. I'm saying you can do both—at the same time.

Exercise is not something that has to be done every day, and if you miss a day, please don't kick yourself for it. Some days you either don't have the time or feel too lousy. Recently, I injured my foot and was feeling very glum about not exercising, especially walking in place. How silly, I thought! I was beating myself up for doing what I was supposed to do, resting my foot. Sometimes, exercise can make you feel so good it becomes addicting, and when you miss it, you feel down and guilty. You crave the release and high you get from it. While that's a perfectly wonderful thing (there are worse thing you could be addicted to), there are going to be times you need a break for whatever reason. It's important to realize it's okay, and you can get back into whatever kind of routine you're comfortable with when the time's right. Also, when my foot was injured, I could still do deep breathing exercises, stretches on the floor, and meditations.

Remember, a little exercise is so much better than none at all. Take things one day, or one step, at a time and always feel good about what you've accomplished. You deserve it.

Although I don't have one, I'd love a treadmill. If you have one that's sitting around collecting dust or serving as a place to hang your laundry, perhaps it's time you give that a try. Don't push yourself, and remember, you can watch your favorite television while you're doing it.

I have this wonderful stretchy band I use when I exercise. It's great for toning muscles, and the act of stretching the band out and returning to the original position, relieves tension in my muscles. If you had time to do that alone for ten minutes a day (you can even do it with a huge, thick rubber band), your mind focuses on the band (not your pain), and you still get the same sense of accomplishment and stress relief as with the other exercises mentioned (not to mention nicely toned arms and legs, depending on how you use it).

When I'm going full throttle cleaning the house, I sometimes consider that to be my exercise for the day. You burn a lot of calories when you clean, and again, your mind is taken from your emotions and channeled into something positive. When it's heavy cleaning time, I dive in, get 'into it,' and something drives me to keep going. When I get to the point where I've worked up a sweat, I know I'm getting a good workout. Typically, I'm exhausted by the time I'm done, and I don't feel one ounce of 'guilt' for not having done one of my routines.

Exercise doesn't always have to be something that's fast, raising your heart rate. One of the most relaxing and challenging forms of exercise are yoga and Tai Chi. When I feel like breaking things up a bit, I'll grab my yoga mat and/or yoga ball, and practice yoga. Although I'm not very good at it, I love it and the way it quickly reduces stress. So what if I'm not walking around, stretching a band, lifting weights, or using a treadmill? Yoga cleanses the mind, forces you to focus on what you're trying to achieve (focus, balance, coordination, positions, etc.), and is like meditation in motion. Yoga tones, makes me more agile, keeps my emotions in check by freeing my mind, in turn reducing my stress level. Believe me when I say I'm a beginner at yoga. I don't do it enough to be anything but. So what? If it makes me feel better, it doesn't matter what level I'm at. I'm not exercising for anyone but me and am not out to impress anyone. What matters most is how much exercise helps me and can help you when you feel you're ready to give it a try.

Remember, there's no particular form of exercise I advocate because we're all different. Also, I'm not qualified to say what's best for you. That's between you and your doctor. It's up to you to decide what kind of exercise you like, when you want to do it, and how often. If you think you can't do it right now, that's okay. The only thing I'll interject is this: If you're really stuck in an emotional rut and can't seem to find a way out, exercise, even a little, will help you feel better. Plain and simple. As always, check with your doctor first.

Finding Your Creative Self—
Where's Your Music?

Creativity is our souls' way of expressing who we really are, and there are countless ways to be creative. When you allow yourself to be creative, your mind is taken away from everything else except for where your passion lies. Whether it's cooking, drawing, decorating, singing, sewing, knitting...being creative is like a form of meditation. By focusing on one thing, your entire being enters a different state—a state of relaxation and calm. Example: When I play the piano and sing, I'm transported into another place—that of my true self. My entire world changes. I'm not thinking about my miscarriage, the dishes that need to be done, the rugs that need vacuuming, the trash that needs to go out, the argument I just had, the worries of today and the future. The only thing that matters when I play the piano and sing is playing the piano and singing. My mind is given the rest it needs. I am taken away from the external and brought into the internal—me. Whether you're married, single, partnered, have children or don't, or are in a demanding job—you are still you and, we all have a creative essence about us. It's the seed planted in our souls before reaching this earth. It's the gift you've been given by God, if you will, to be used, enjoyed, and shared with others. There's a part of each of us that cannot and should not be identified with what we do, have or who we're with. While those things may hold great value, they don't define you. When you stand apart from all that is your life and all that is external to your life, look yourself in the mirror and ask: Who am I? What are my dreams? What to I love to do? What have I not done in years, but wish I could? What part of me isn't getting the attention it deserves? I understand that time is precious— but so are you. Finding the time, even if only a little here and there to nurture your creative self is worth it because you are. What you loved and dreamed of as a little girl—art, music, writing, dance, whatever—lies buried under the 'grown up world' and all its expectations. The key is, your creative self is still there, you just forgot who she is. If you feel you're simply not a creative person, please allow yourself the chance to discover and unearth your own, unique, creative self. She's there...believe me.

"I don't have a creative bone in my body." I've heard that so many times, and while the person thinks it's true, I don't. I'm a singer, pianist, poet, writer. While I was singing in a band, so many people told me how lucky I was, and that they "couldn't sing a note." Okay. Perhaps they weren't singers—but, I'm sure they had creative talents in other areas. To be creative doesn't mean you have to be into 'the arts.' That's bologna. I am not a painter, sculptor, cannot knit, don't have a clue about sewing, am not an interior decorator, gardener, etc. There are literally thousands of things that make a person creative, perhaps more. So, before you go and mumble to yourself that you can't possibly be creative, please stick with me.

On many occasions I've wandered through shops, admiring the handmade jewelry, beautifully knitted blankets and scarves, pottery, dried flowers and wreaths, candles and more. Behind each one of those items is a person. That individual found their creative self and ran with it.

My sister is an excellent gardener. She loves planting flowers, etc., and unlike mine, they don't die. She arranges them without much thought—it's a talent she's been blessed with. She's also a wonderful fitness instructor and personal trainer. When someone is bored with a routine, she knows how to vary it to make it interesting again. Additionally, she's an excellent cartoonist. No one taught her—she found it herself, nurtured it, and developed her talent over the years.

My other sister has a knack for fixing little things like a broken clasp on a necklace, knowing what wallpaper would look best in a room and hanging it herself. She'll see a piece of 'junk' furniture and transform it into something beautiful. She knows how to create arts and crafts projects for children and is a wonderful teacher. She's also a great cook.

When I was a little girl, my mother decided to paint a mural on the bathroom wall. She probably figured, "What do I have to lose? It looks like hell anyway." So, fearlessly, she bought the paint, taught herself how to 'do' trees, and created a mural of frogs on a lake, swimming, resting on lily pads, relaxing under trees. The water reflects the blue sky, the trees provide ample shade for the frogs, the sunlight cascades down upon the middle of the pond—and she did it without *ever* having done anything like it before. My mother discovered that part of her creative self—and took a chance. In retrospect, she most likely did it because the three of us girls were driving her crazy and she needed some 'me' time! How relaxing it must have been to focus on nothing but her mural for a while. What a feeling of accomplishment she must have had when it was complete.

My best friend loves to draw, is an excellent poet, a wonderful writer, a dynamite cook, terrific at making crafts, and loves to attempt new things all the time, whether she knows how or not. She jumps right in.

Another best friend doesn't realize how creative she is. She's always had a beautiful singing voice and is a fantastic writer.

I have a friend who owns a store. She has an uncanny knack of knowing how to create beautiful window displays and amazing in-store displays. She coordinates everything perfectly, always has soothing music playing in the background, could envision what paint colors would be perfect for her new location. Amazing.

Perhaps you're one of those people I often ran into who said, "Gee, I'd love to be able to sing. I've got no talent at all." Hogwash! Do you see how being creative doesn't have to equate to being a singer, actor, painter, etc.?

So, where's your creativity? Do you have a liking for beads? Maybe you should give it a whirl and try making some beaded necklaces or bracelets. Perhaps you've always loved pottery. Is there a place nearby where you could take a class? You could be a master potter and not realize it! Find yourself doodling a lot? Who knows? You could be more than a doodler if you dove into it and tried. Are you good at planning parties? That's a talent. When you do it for a living they call you an Event Planner. Is there a story inside of you waiting to get out? Maybe it's supposed to get out, and you simply need to write. You'll never know if you don't try.

Making clothes, knitting, crocheting, gardening, cooking, baking, decorating, making candles, painting, restoring furniture, making baskets, writing children's stories, scrap-booking and rubber-stamping, trying your hand at a musical instrument, tinkering around with things that are broken, wood carving, writing Santa letters to kids, getting involved in your community, buying some silk or dried flowers to arrange, making little signs to hang on front doors welcoming people, planting tulips, trees, roses, giving a chair an antique finish, repainting your living room, needlework, poetry, making your own greeting cards, helping to plan a friend's wedding, making ponytail holders with elastics and buttons, and countless other activities comprise creativity. You don't have to be the best at it—it's finding what you like and doing it that counts.

Why? Because when you use your creative self, you're nurturing your soul. You're giving your mind a complete break from the day's thoughts, pressures, emotions, worries, and focusing on one thing. Finding your creative self is like discovering a piece to a puzzle you never knew existed. When you decide to try your hands, or voice, whatever— at something, in a sense you're meditating. Focusing on one thing (like the word *om* when you meditate) is relaxing, fulfilling, and leaves you feeling more connected to the real you. By the real you I mean the person you were when the days were carefree. That little girl who loved to dress her dolls up, or play with Hot-Wheels in the dirt, or climb trees, or color for hours. When you tap into your creative self, you find that little girl again, except now she's all grown up and instead of dressing her dolls, she's making clothes. Instead of playing with Hot-Wheels, she's restoring an old car. Instead of coloring in a book, she's painting a mural on her bathroom wall. Instead of climbing trees, she's climbing ladders to pick apples from the tree she planted. Instead of using her mother's makeup, she's applying makeup on her friend so she looks perfect for a big night out. Instead of inviting her girlfriends over for a tea-party, she's planning a party for herself or someone else. Instead of making a bowl out of popsicle sticks, she's making a designer lamp out of bark and twigs. Instead of painting her mother's walls and getting into trouble, she's stenciling borders on her living room wall, making them warm and inviting. Instead of being the leader in a game of street hockey, she's helping the elderly exercise. Instead of playing with her mother's thread, she's creating beautiful needlework.

I could keep going, but think you get the idea. Creativity is not limited. If you haven't found your creative self, or think one doesn't exist, please rethink that. We all have gifts and talents—some are simply undiscovered.

When I was a little girl, I'd go downstairs into the playroom, go through my parents old forty-fives, put one on the record player, and sing. I'd do it for hours and never tire. I remember *not* thinking about anything else and how naturally it came.

As we grow up, we live, learn, feel joy and pain, and somewhere beneath all the rubble, our creative self lies waiting to burst free.

Let her out.

Being creative is like a great therapy session without a time limit or a hefty price tag. That's not a knock to therapists—it's a point. When I'm feeling wound up, you know what I do? I either play my keyboard and sing, use my new karaoke machine and sing some more, take a trip to the music studio where my parents teach so I can play a beautiful grand piano for a while, write some poetry, try something new with throws or pillows in the living room—just to name a few. When I submerge myself in my creativity, my muscles automatically loosen, my chest opens up and I breathe easier, my tears dry up, my heart slows down a bit, my headache goes away, my sour mood evaporates, my negative thinking comes to a halt, my feelings of hopelessness dissipate, my cabin fever takes a back seat, and I feel like *me* again. The me I want to feel like. That's how much finding your creativity can do for you—without a pill, a doctor's bill, or anything else. All you need is *you.*

If you see yourself as black and white, dull, without a creative bone in your body, you're wrong. You are a rainbow of color, a unique woman with so much to offer yourself, those around you, and the world, through your creativity. Once you find it, you'll never see the world, or yourself, the same way. It's like a window opened that's been stuck shut for years.

In being creative you will derive: inner peace, inner calm, and inner joy. I know you don't have all day to use your creative self, but think of the possibilities of what an hour here or there can do for you. Allow yourself to escape from life's demands for a while. Allow yourself to not feel sad for a while. Allow yourself to express for a while.

Allow yourself to be you.

Stuck on finding that creative you? Here's a way to do it:

1. Write down ten things you like. It doesn't matter what they are, just write them and don't think about it.

2. Next, write down *why* you like those things. It doesn't have to be long. For example: You wrote down candles. Why do you like candles? Let's say you wrote: I love the scent. I like the way they look. Candles relax me.

3. After you've written down all the whys, pick one of your ideas and see where you could run with it. For example: Candles. You like them because of the scent, the look, and their relaxing qualities. Now it's time to explore. Do you think you'd like to try your hand at making candles? All you have to do is go to a craft supply store, get a book, some basic candlemaking supplies, and try it. If you're a real candle lover, imagine the satisfaction you'd get from making your very own, in your favorite scents. Think about how relaxed you'd feel while making them, and the wonderful anticipation you'd feel waiting for your first one to be done. If it's something you really love, you could make candles as gifts for people, to sell at a craft fair or bazaar, or perhaps in a gift shop. Not only would you be tapping into your creative self, you could make some money at the same time!

If you follow this simple formula: Write down ten things you love, why, and what you could do with that 'thing'—you're bound to find part of your creative self. There may be more than one thing on your list that you can explore—and that's super!

Where's Your Music?

"It is sad that so many people will die with their music still inside of them."

That is I quote a recently heard on a television show. I am not sure who it belongs to, but its words hold a powerful message. I know they had quite an impact on me.

Where is your music? It can be anything you love. Are you doing what you want with your life, or are you living half the life you want to? Does your heart sing each and every day because you are doing what you love or do you wake feeling like part of you is missing? Or, that you're somehow incomplete?

I know that it might be impossible to be a famous driver with NASCAR, or a singer cutting CD's, getting loads of air time and signing autographs.

But, are you doing what you love on some level?

We all have gifts. Some of us are musical; some are great teachers; some are artists; some are wonderful parents; some are mechanically inclined; some are great with plants; some are compassionate; some are writers; some are speakers; and so much more.

If you search your heart and still yourself, you will know what it is that you love. If it's missing from your life, you will know that, too. For there is a spot in each and every one of us that can only be filled by doing what we are meant to do.

And we feel the emptiness when it's there.

Let's say that you quiet yourself and you start thinking about children. You may or may not have some of your own, but for some reason your thoughts keep going to them. You've always loved them. Maybe your thoughts lean towards disabled children. It's quite possible that you've always been a wonderful helper and giver. You may be a terrific parent. But, if you don't feel complete, in this scenario, think about the possibility that you would love to be around more children. Maybe you'd be a great teacher. Or, if you don't have the education to be a teacher, maybe you could be an assistant someplace or even donate some time to helping children in some way. If you could get your degree, then maybe that's what you should do. It's possible that you were meant to start a youth group in your city or town to provide laughter, hope, and light to the young ones. The possibilities are endless.

I have stilled myself quite often and have heard my heart speak to me. It tells me that I love to give to people. I love to make them feel, whether it's through writing or singing. I know that I have not even come close to my full potential and that there's much more that I want to explore and do in these areas. I know that I was extremely satisfied when I sang in a band. Not only was I doing something that I loved, but I was around so much positive energy. It's as if the music created a bond between myself and the crowd, and that connection, that rare moment when you are relating to people on a spiritual level, is precious. Since I have stopped doing that, I know that it's a piece of my life that's like a missing part of a puzzle.

So, I must think of a way to incorporate that back into my life because I know that it is part of what my purpose is. Without it, there is an emptiness deep inside. I am not willing to sit on the sidelines of my life and forever feel like part of me is missing. It may not be joining a band again, but music, in some way, will be shared by me with others. Maybe it will be helping to entertain in local schools or nursing homes. It's not the same as a night club, but I don't need the night club. I need to reach people, and that can be done anywhere.

Do you know where your music is? More importantly, do you know what your music is?

Don't be one of those people who leaves this earth with their music still inside of them. You deserve to experience the delight, we all do, of 'singing your song,' no matter what it may be.

Journaling Your Way to Emotional Release

I write and I write and I write when I'm feeling happy, down, sad, confused, disappointed, joyful, fearful…I write because it allows me to vent, and I often gain a better understanding of myself through my own words. I write because I need to let who I am and what I'm feeling out. Sometimes I cry when I write, other times I smile. Sometimes I feel very connected to God when I write; other times I simply feel connected to me. There are times my writing points out my strengths, and others when it points out my weaknesses. Writing serves to make me appreciate the small, often overlooked beautiful things in life, and those feelings carry themselves from my notebook into my life. My writing is sometimes nothing but scribble, but the scribble means something. Sometimes an unexpected poem jumps from my pen to the paper, and I read it in amazement because it was so unplanned—so 'fly by the seat of my pants.' Writing, or journaling, has enabled me to see more clearly who I am, what I need, feel, want, or must change. Writing has served as an emotional release when I feel there's none—all it takes is an open mind, a pen, and some paper. The benefits are worth more than gold. Finding yourself is a great treasure, a constant journey, and requires only one thing: you and your desire to get to the heart of whatever it is you need to discover. Writing can be your tool, your key to unlocking the door to your soul. Writing can dry tears, create smiles, open doors, make you see things that were right under your nose. Writing will take you on an incredible journey: the journey to your incredible self.

Years ago people referred to a journal as a diary. With the advent of the Internet, people are journaling online, learning how to write their life stories, etc. For our purposes, let's say you're journaling at home, either typing on your computer or writing by hand. Your journal is for you—where you later take it is your decision.

I've always found that when I'm stuck for the right words, or can't express my feelings verbally, writing has been the perfect outlet. Since I was a teenager, I've used writing to express my deepest feelings. When I was a teenager, my father and I were like oil and water for a brief time. Oh, it was awful! Thank God it didn't last. However, during that time, I'd sometimes end up writing my feelings down on paper and giving them to my Dad. He often started this process by writing me a letter, which explains how genetics will run their course. Later, I wrote myself through feelings of a first love, fears, concerns, excitement, getting married, and writing really became an outlet after I miscarried. I wrote poetry, a song dedicated to my lost baby, and wrote through all the feelings I couldn't articulate. Writing also served as an invaluable tool in getting me through both my anxiety attacks and my divorce. Whenever something doesn't feel right in my life—I write. Often, I gain a better understanding of how I truly feel after reading my own words and experience a sensation of emotional purging when I'm done. It's like I've carried a huge weight upon my chest, and after writing about whatever I'm feeling, most of it, if not all, is lifted.

When I first began *I Never Held You,* it was journaling in a way. I knew I had to write—it was a feeling I couldn't shake. There was so much I had to say, to you, to myself, to all women who miscarried. The idea of it being a book came later; although, from the start I believed that if I could somehow help through my words, I'd find a way to do it. I was passionate about it, and still am.

Some of the poems and pages of emotions I still have following my miscarriage are heartbreaking. But, they served a very important purpose. I felt so alone and misunderstood that I had to write. It was my way of making my emotions clear—to myself. It was so difficult to explain to someone everything that was running through me. But, when I was alone with nothing but a pen and paper, everything inside spilled out onto those blank sheets. I'd read them afterwards and feel a sense of calm, even if I sometimes cried while reading them.

When I think about it, I've been journaling ever since I can remember. As an adult, it became more prevalent. Much good has come as a result, both personally and professionally. Had I not written so much about my anxiety attacks I never would have been published in a book about anxiety. Had I not written so much about my feelings in the form of poetry, I wouldn't have the published egreetings online, or have work published with a major greeting card publisher. Had I not written so much about my faith, I wouldn't have been published in a very popular inspirational series of books. Had I not written about my miscarriage and *all* the feelings associated with it, I wouldn't be sitting her right now writing this book.

After all is said and done, journaling has opened two very important doors for me: the door to my soul and the door to opportunity. While writing, the door to opportunity was the last thing on my mind, but it came later—after the emotional release was felt, after I'd come to terms with whatever I was experiencing. It was at that point, I allowed my thoughts to be shared and the doors flew open.

Whether or not you decide to take your private self and share it is your choice. It's not paramount to journaling. The goal of writing down your feelings is this: to gain a better understanding of yourself, and to release unexplained, unidentified emotions onto paper (or computer screen). You will gain tremendous relief from the process of journaling, and it will help you in your overall healing process. The better you understand *what* it is you're feeling, the better able you are to cope with it. Writing is often the equivalent of finding the needle in the haystack. When everything verbal fails you, your heart and soul never will when you allow them to come out privately onto paper.

Don't worry about format, spelling, technique, etc. None of that matters. None of that will make you feel better—so toss the idea that you're not a writer out the window. Just write—that's all you need to do. Not for an audience, but for your very special, remarkable self who needs to express and understand herself better.

Just take it a word at a time.

Examples from my life's journaling:

Here's a song I wrote about my baby after I miscarried. In all of these examples, I needed to let out powerful emotions. I didn't know what I was going to write, I simply wrote. Sometimes, it came out in the form of a song, other times, just feelings. Many times, my feelings came out as poems. I doesn't matter what form your feelings take, as long as they are set free.

Angel Wings

At the ending of the day when I'm weary
after a waterfall of tears have all been cried—
and I'm feeling like the skies will always be dreary—
nothing's there to fill the emptiness inside.

I lay my head upon my favorite pillow
just close my eyes to block all the sorrow—
wonderin' where I'll ever find the strength inside—
to do it all again—tomorrow.
And then I feel it—

inside me.
I feel it—
around me.
Like a gentle hand just wiped away the tears—
and held me close to wash away my fears.

It's you, my angel, watching over me.
And I know no matter what tomorrow brings,
You'll be here to wrap me in your angel wings—
your lovin' angel wings.

The sun comes up, it's time to face the day
and I think that things are going to be all right—
But as the day wears on my nerves begin to fray—
I feel the hollowness that creeps in every night.

And like clockwork all the tears begin to fall
As I look at my reflection in the glass—
the eyes looking back at me make me feel small—
and I ask, my God, how long's this going to last?

And then I feel it—
inside me.
I feel it—
around me.
Like a gentle hand just wiped away the tears—
and held me close to wash away my fears.

It's you, my angel, watching over me.
And I know no matter what tomorrow brings,
You'll be here to wrap me in your angel wings—
your lovin' angel wings. (Thank God for your angel wings)

May, 2003 (Even though it's been fifteen years since my miscarriage, I still think about it, because I don't have a child and long for one so much. Here's an example of journaling where I simply wrote a letter to God.)

Dear God,
Why Can't I be a Mother?
Mother's Day nears, and I thank you, God, for my Mother. She is love. She is beauty. She is strength and dignity. She is my anchor. She is

a gift from You.

And then, swelling up over the wall comes a wave of tears, making me feel ungrateful and selfish. I have been blessed. A wonderful family surrounds me, loves me, appreciates me. I know these things—yet the wave overpowers genuine gratitude, washing it out to sea.

I am drowning in my own sea of tears, feeling the emptiness of a black hole which remains in my gut. A black hole within my womb, unfilled by a child—once was, but never to fruition.

My baby is in heaven—never seen, never held by me, but mine. "I love you," I whisper.

Mothers walking children in strollers down the street are like daggers to my heart and I feel ashamed. Celebrate their joy, I repeat over and over. Don't be jealous, it's a sin.

Yet, I am jealous. I am unbelievably jealous and hate myself for it. Do they know how blessed they are? Do they know how You, God, have given them the most precious gift in the world? Do they know my heart screams to have a baby fall asleep upon my chest to the rhythm of blended heartbeats?

Another year, another Mother's Day, another 'vacant' sign on the door to my soul. I loathe my self pity, but it's stuck to me like gum on a shoe.

I love my nieces and nephews. They are beautiful, and I find comfort knowing they are a small part of me, too. I am happy for my family, who now have families of their own. They've done a wonderful job. They are beautiful people. Beautiful Mothers, just like our own. I thank them for giving me such wonderful children to love and call family.

I wish I could have done the same for them. Always an Aunt, never a Mother.

That's okay, I repeat over and over. Don't be such an ungrateful, selfish woman. I want to scold myself for thinking about what I don't have instead of what I do. If I were to look into Your eyes, I would feel ashamed and unworthy—completely devoid of true faith.

Should I apologize for wanting to be called Mother? Should I feel guilty for what my heart naturally cries for? Can I turn off the need, the longing, the hope? If I'm not to be a Mother, why was I born with an instinct to become one? Why wasn't I born one of those women who don't want children? Wouldn't it have been easier?

No one said it would be easy. Guess what? It's not.

Along with Mother's Day, another birthday will arrive for me this month. Another year's gone by full of new things, and full of the same heavy bags of emptiness I carry. Couldn't dump them off, again.

Couldn't let go of the dream. Couldn't let go and let You, God.

Soon, my body will say it's no longer a remote possibility. Nature will have control over my fate, not I. You've built me to shut down, and that's what I'll do. My womb will state to me that it's no longer capable of carrying a child because my body won't be able to make one. Maybe then it'll be easier because this 'biological' clock that keeps ticking louder and louder will shut *up!*

Perhaps not. My heart's told me since I was a little girl that I wanted to adopt a little girl—or boy. Some call it the adoption gene—and if there's such a thing, I was born with it. My life would feel so incredibly complete if I could shower my love upon a child who has no one to love him or her. I don't need to bear a child to feel like a Mother. I just need to love a child to feel like a Mother. Blood isn't the answer. Love is. If You, God, see fit that I become a Mother and bring a child into my heart, I will know that child is truly mine because You intended it to be that way.

If not, I will know for reasons unknown to me that it wasn't in Your plan. Not on my map through this life. I may not like it, but have to accept it.

And my human self still screams inside. I can talk about Your plan all I want, and believe what I'm saying. I can even take comfort in it, but it doesn't stop the wave from crashing. It doesn't stop me from feeling. It doesn't stop the tears from flowing. It doesn't stop me from whispering in the dark of night, "Why can't I be a Mother?"

Do you see the intensity of my feelings? In one example, they came out in the form of a song— one that's sad yet hopeful. In the other, my feelings of longing were so pronounced that if I didn't write about them, I'd pop. So, in the above example, I wrote a letter to God and basically spilled my guts. In the end, I learned more about myself, my real needs, and my soul through writing. I hope you're able to do the same and open yourself up to more positive things coming to you by purging your sad or negative thoughts onto paper. It truly is a cleansing experience.

I don't have the television as a platform to help balance the scales by providing some light and love in His name to all, but I have my words. And so, I'll use them, praying that they will touch the hearts and souls of those who need to be reminded that: *You* are not alone, *you* never will be— God is beside *you* in all ways for all days.

God Bless *you,* Your Angel Baby, the USA, and *the world.*

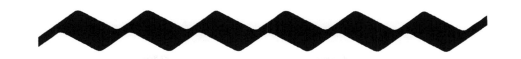

Part Three

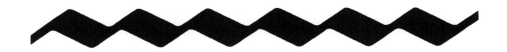

Thoughts to Ponder

Thoughts on Friendship

Friends are your greatest asset—no matter how you feel, up or down, they love you anyway. I recently read this on a coffee mug: "Friends are like thighs—always sticking together." They are there for you, and you for them. They tell us we are not going crazy and bring us back to ourselves. Friends are such an incredible gift. In allowing your heart to open up to them, they open up to you. Bonds are formed which override the boundaries of time and distance. Friendship endures all, and when it's from the heart, can withstand any test of time. I thank God for my friends. They are my certainty when I'm unsure, my laughter amidst tears, my hope when all seems dark.

The Screaming Baby

My best friend had just had her first baby. She was newly married, and her husband worked third shift which meant that she was up all day with the baby while he slept and all night while he worked.

One evening she called me. She sounded half out of her mind. I could hear the baby, my Goddaughter, screaming as she usually did, in the background. Being a new mother, she was exhausted and absolutely beside herself. There was nothing she could do to stop the her from screaming, and in sheer desperation she asked me to come over for fear that she'd go crazy.

"I'm going to throw her out the window if she doesn't stop!"

Of course, she didn't mean that literally. She was and is one of the best mothers I know. But, she was at her wit's end.

I hopped in my car and drove quickly to her house. Fortunately, she was only ten minutes away. I didn't know much about babies, but I knew a lot about my best friend. She never asked for anything—so I knew this was serious.

I walked into the apartment and could hear my Goddaughter wailing at the top of her precious lungs. It was bed time, and she never liked to go to sleep. It was as if she thought she'd miss something.

My best friend looked worn and exasperated, and my heart went out to her. I told her to give me the baby and sit and relax. She hadn't gotten any sleep, and I, naively thinking I could get any situation under control, figured I'd rock the baby for a while and they'd both get a good night's rest.

I'd feel like a hero.

Reality didn't take long to strike. After about ten minutes of relentless screaming I realized that I couldn't get her to quiet down, either. I felt my head start to throb and my jaw clench. All the feelings of frustration that my girlfriend had I was having.

The only difference was, I could go home.

I rocked her. I stood up and walked. I talked soothingly to her. Nothing worked.

Who was I to think that I could do any better than her own mother? Boy, was I wrong.

I looked at my best friend who was sprawled out on the chair, eyes half open and said, "I'm going to throw her out the window! Oh my God, I don't know how you can take this!"

Of course, I didn't mean that literally, either. But, I could see how rattled a new mother could get after that experience.

Suddenly, my best friend smiled. Then she laughed. It was so wonderful to see her expression change.

"You don't know how good it makes me feel to hear you say that. I thought I was going crazy."

We both laughed, while the baby continued to scream.

I stayed over that night, and we endured the screaming baby for several more hours. Finally, she fell asleep. It was probably two or three in the morning.

Enjoying the silence, we both sat in the living room drinking coffee and talking. Make that whispering. We didn't want to take any chances.

Sometime around dawn, she went to bed and I fell asleep on the couch. After only a few hours of sleep, I heard it.

The screaming baby.

My friend had already gotten her and was out in the kitchen feeding her. I kissed the baby good morning, and my friend and I chuckled. At least she'd gotten some sleep.

I offered to stick around so that she could enjoy one of the many things those of us who have no children take for granted—a well deserved shower. Unless her husband was home and awake, she didn't get that luxury and had to squeeze quick ones in during the scant time he was there so that he could watch the baby.

I told her to take her time.

As I sat with my Goddaughter in my arms, watching her peacefully drink from her bottle, I smiled. She was so beautiful, so incredibly precious, and so unbelievably loud when she wanted to be!

My friend came into the living room looking refreshed and rejuvenated. I felt happy for her. She needed the time to take her time, and I was glad to be there so she could have it.

To this day, nearly seventeen years later, we both remember that night. We both learned something. I learned how difficult it can be to be a new mother who's alone and tired. She learned that she was not crazy. She was just tired.

We still reflect back on it and laugh. It's one of many wonderful pages we have in the book of our friendship.

Over the years, the tides have turned in both of our lives, and we have been there for one another. She's seen me through the loss of a pregnancy, and I hers. She was there for me when I went through the trauma of a divorce, and she helped me with my subsequent anxiety attacks. I was there for her when she experienced panic attacks after a nearly fatal auto accident with her children in the car. She was the one who got me to eat, even if slowly, when I felt I couldn't. I was there when her third born son was in Boston with a tumor on his heart, praying for her and standing beside her. I was there when she buried her mother far too soon, and she was there when I buried both of my grandparents, even though she wasn't feeling well. She has supported me in my music and in my writing, and I have done the same for her.

From the day we met in high school, something between us "clicked." It was as if God put her on this earth to be my best friend, and I am here as hers. It's hard to believe that so many years have gone by. I'm thirty-five now, and as I reflect over the hills and valleys of our lives, I can see that we have shared in those times together. If not together physically, our hearts are forever bonded, and we are there for one another always in thought and spirit.

There are many acquaintances you make in life, but there are just a few true, wonderful friends who bless your life forever.

I am so thankful and always will be for our friendship. I know that we will be writing many more pages to the book of our lives: some happy, some sad, but all creating a beautiful story of trust, honesty, and love. The meaning of friendship itself.

Thoughts on Heaven: Questions to David

We all have different ideas of what heaven is, and some of you may question whether there is a heaven. Personally, my belief in heaven is what carried me through not only my miscarriage, but through other very trying times in my life. Knowing in my heart that the baby I never held resides in a world much more beautiful than this one still provides me with great comfort today, and also makes me keenly aware of my connection to my baby. One of my best friends, Nancy, once said to me, "You know, Ellen, you're still a mother. No one can take that away from you. Your baby lives on in heaven, and knows you are his mother."

You can't imagine the comfort I took in her words! I already believed in heaven, and in a God that is the creator of everything and everyone on this planet. I knew my baby was in His kingdom, but to actually have my friend say it just the way she did made my heart sing— and yes, my eyes water. Such validation flowed through me, such hope that one day I would hold the baby I never held.

Whatever your particular thoughts are on God, heaven, faith, please read the following with an open mind and take it how you will. I'm not forcing my beliefs on you, but I thought it was important to share a very surreal experience I had one day while sitting in front of the very computer I'm in front of now.

My life was forever changed the day I had a conversation with the brother I never knew, but always felt connected to.

I am of the earthly plane; living out my life, trying to find my path and learning on my journey. I believe that God, the Universal Power, is there all the time as are spirit beings and angels, always looking after me and trying to help where they can.

There are those we have loved and lost who are no longer of this world, but of another. I feel in my heart it is just as real as the one I know, possibly more so.

When my mother was seven months pregnant with me, she buried a son. His name was David. I never knew him as we here on earth define 'knowing'; yet somewhere within me there has always been a connection to him. It's quite difficult to explain. I can only say that throughout my entire life I have felt that his presence and his life, although short here on earth, have touched mine in ways that I cannot describe nor understand.

I just know that he is there, and that we are still sister and brother.

My mother kissed a new life hello and another goodnight. When I say that I somehow felt some of her pain while in her womb as she and my father buried their son may lead some of you to come to the conclusion that I am not 'all there.' That is up to you, but I ask you to keep an open mind when dealing with the unknown and know, too, that those who know me well would call me anything but 'insane.'

Something compelled me to have a conversation with David, my brother, and ask him some questions about his life. I am not gifted in contacting the spirit world; these are simply thoughts that came to me, like that of a radio frequency, and I am writing them down. You may call it a writer's overactive imagination or you may attribute it to something more concrete than that. I just know that there are feelings or hunches that are so strong you cannot disregard them. It may be a doorway has been opened to those in the spirit world because I have allowed it to be opened. I believe and am receptive. I think it is beyond my earthly understanding. We create earthly laws, judgments, stigmas, rules, and beliefs. They are not created by God; therefore, we cannot understand what we simply do not know of another realm, another world. A world much closer to God, the Universal Life Force.

I want you to know that as I typed this, I just let my fingers do the walking after I asked a question. No thought as to grammar or style came from me. The words seemed to pop into my head, and I typed them down as they came. It was even faster than that.

Me: David, I have always thought about you. I have wondered what you would have been like if you remained here on earth, and I have felt something very special towards you since I can remember. I've always had a curiosity about you, and want to know if you know me and watch over me here on earth.

David: Yes, Ellen, you are my sister. I have known you for your entire life and I do, indeed watch over you and your other sisters. I also watch over Mom and Dad. I Love them very much and I love you, too, very much. I want you to know that when you feel me near, it is because I am near. Although I have resumed a life here, in what you call 'Heaven,' I am able to see and feel what goes on on the earth and am acutely aware of what your feelings are, be they sadness, joy, guilt, depression, happiness or fear. One thing I will say is that I wish you wouldn't waste so much time being afraid. For, where you are and what you are experiencing are only a fraction of what is to come. Your life, as you know it now, is quite short compared to the life that lies ahead for you. You are on earth to learn and you are learning quite a bit. Keep your mind and heart open and listen to your instincts. Often times, they are us, and what I mean by us is a group of spirits as you call us, trying to help you and yes, we listen to your prayers for help and those of thanks.

Me: David, why did God take you away so early? You were not even two and it hurt Mom and Dad very much.

David: I was sent to earth for a very short time for a reason. Whenever tragedy strikes, people blame God for it. It's not God's fault, it's all in the plan. I could go into greater detail here about the plan, but I think it would be too complex right now. Let me just say this, that there is always pain in life and without it you would not know joy. There are always lessons to be taught and although I was not on the earthly plane for a very long time, at least in earthly time, I taught a lesson through the pain of loss. I know it's hard for you to understand, but I want you to know that it was not God's intention to hurt your parents when I left to come back home. It was to make them into the people that they are today. They are strong and they appreciate life so very much. They have been an inspiration to many and they are great teachers. Your mother, although appearing like a rock, felt tremendous pain when she lost me. So did your father. Your mother has always had a tremendous faith in God and in His plan, and that helped carry her through that most painful time. Your father, on the other hand, had a very difficult time with my passing and over time, he learned to not blame God for the terrible things in life that sometimes happen. For a long time he did that and had very mixed feelings about God and His mercy. I knew that. He suffered very much but look at him now. He is faithful and such a giver. He is a kind, good soul and I am so proud to have been born to both he and your mother. Cherish them, Ellen, like I know you already do. Show it even more. For there will come a time when you feel like you cannot talk to them or show them your love anymore when they leave this earth. Know that you can. They will always be alive and there to listen to you and to love you. There are so many of us that do now.

Me: I sometimes thought that my father wished I was a boy, although he never, ever said that. As a matter of fact, he's told me that all he cared about when I was born was that I was healthy. I believe him, but what do you have to say about that?

David: Your father loves you for who you are and always has. He feels a special connection with you because of the gift of music that you both share. He loves your sisters just as much, but the musical connection that you share with him is special and you should treasure that. It gives you something that's rare and wonderful; an understanding of a part of each other that many don't have. The same goes for your mother. When she told you that she felt there was something special about you when you were born, she meant it. I think you feel what I mean. Your mother loves all three of you girls very much, no more, no less. But, with you and your mother, there is a very spiritual bond that will never be broken and that pleases God very much. You are so special to both of your parents. Please don't ever forget that.

Me: Do you hear me when I ask for help or when I don't ask but feel I need it?

David: I want you to know that you never have to talk for me, or for any other spirits as you call us, to hear you. It's not like on earth. Oh, yes, I know that there are those that claim they can read the minds of others. As a matter of fact, there are people with that gift. But, here, it's so very different from what you know. Here, we just have too think something and it is known. If you think something or feel something I feel it, too. If you are sad I know it and feel it and am there beside you to help get you through, even if you don't ask. But, I want you to be happier. Please hear me. I want you to enjoy life more and to see all the beauty that is around you on the earthly plane. That is very important. You are there to learn and to experience and to use the gifts that God gave you. In many ways, you do, but you, like so many others, have not even come close to your full potential. Pray to God to reach your full potential. Ask Him what He wants you to do and follow his answers. You will live a much more fulfilling life on earth. God wants you to be happy, Ellen. That's all he wants. By following His word you will be. Don't ignore that feeling you get inside that tells you that there's more you want to do with your life. You have a great tendency to want to help people and that is a good thing. You hold yourself back from doing that and that makes me sad, but it makes God sad. Don't ever think He doesn't love you and care for you. Remember, He is your father. Your heavenly Father and just like the 'Dad' that you have on earth, he hurts when you hurt and is happy when you are. Follow your heart. Follow the truth. The truth is God. There is no other truth. It's easy to be fooled. Trust in God and you won't be. You will know you are on the right path for you. The true path. Your true path.

Me: I often talk to people I love who have died, like Grammy, Pop and Nana. Do they hear me, too? Sometimes, I feel my Pop's presence so much it's like he's right beside me. I can even hear his voice sometimes.

David: We are all here watching all of you and loving all of you. Your Pop, (He is smiling now), knows you very well and is always there for you and you are right. You do feel him a lot around you because you ask for him to be near you many times. Especially when you are confused. For in your heart, you know you can turn to him and you take great comfort, as you did when he was alive on the earthly plane, in knowing that he is there—just having him around. He is proud of you but he wants you to know that life has its downs as well as its ups and asks that you not despair so much over certain things and have faith in your plan. If you listen to your heart, which is God, you will be all right. He says, "It's okay, kid."

113

Me: What is it like where you are, in Heaven? Is it like earth? I don't feel it's in the sky, but somehow right here but invisible to me. Maybe it's my imagination or maybe I have read too many books, but something inside of me tells me that where you are is here, just on a different level that I cannot be in or see, but can feel. Is that true?

David: Yes, that's true. When people talk of heaven and they think of it as a place in the sky, that is all that their minds can comprehend. Many think like you do. You are not alone in that thought. And, there is no right or wrong. Whatever people want to feel Heaven is, is okay. Having faith that there is another life and in God is what's really important. Think of Heaven as the earth as you know it, but many, many, many more times as beautiful. It truly is another world, another realm, one that is much easier to live in than where you are now. Here, you don't experience the pain and the lessons that you do on earth, or the earthly plane as you call it. Here, there is Love and Love is God. Here, we can see our lives on earth and we know what we were supposed to have learned or taught and we live for many different reasons than you do. We are not concerned with money or fancy houses or cars or status. For we are all one. We are all a part of God, just like you are on the earthly plane, but we know it here. There is no doubt. We are close to God and He is the Divine and we do not question Him or anything else here. We will never know as much as God, but we have a much greater understanding of His eternal love and we do not live with the fear of death, for we already know that it does not exist. You, not matter how strong your faith, still have a question or a fear about death. I know it because I know your mind and your heart. You have come a long way, but please believe, as I am communicating with you now, that your life on earth is just one life, not the eternal life. It is a place to learn. When you move on to your new and beautiful life, you will know what I mean. Right now, do your best to have the faith that you need and do your best to grasp what I am telling you. You cannot have all the answers now. That would defeat your purpose of being on the earthly plane. Even we don't have all the answers here, but I cannot explain all of that to you right know because I know that you will not understand all of it. It's not that you don't have the intellect, you do. You all do on earth. But, you think a certain way there and in some ways, it's like we are speaking a different language at times. But, we can communicate in the same language, as we are now, in thought, in love, in spirit and in the light of God.

Me: David, I love you and I want you to know that. I've never done anything like this before. I love my family who is there and I want them to know it. I miss them very much but I do believe they are in a better place and that they do live on. Please tell them for me.

David: They already know. And, I love you, too, Ellen. So does God. He is always here for you and so are we, watching you and your sisters and the new baby and everyone. We are here and we listen. Don't be afraid. There is no dark, only if you create it. There is only light, one light, and that's the light of God. Live in that light and you will feel and see things that you never dreamed possible. Live in Love. Know that my love follows you wherever you are and that I and others are always in your heart. Your soul, where God resides, is always with you to help you, give you strength, comfort you and guide you. You have a wonderful soul. All souls are created by God, therefore, they are all wonderful. Sometimes people do bad things, but that is not God's will. That is their will. Walk in light and carry my love for you with you always. Carry God's love with you always.

Me: Thank you, David.

David: You don't have to thank me. There is no need for thanks. There is no need to thank someone for loving you. Just as you are.

Thoughts on Children: Madeline

After my miscarriage, I tended to avoid children. It wasn't done intentionally, but it was so painful so see a woman with her new baby, a pregnant woman, a mother walking her baby down the street. I could barely get through the grocery store without losing it every time I found myself passing the baby isle! God, it was awful. It felt like there was no escaping the pain. Then, my sister had a baby. Well, I couldn't avoid my sister or the baby! I didn't want to. My niece, Madeline, has brought so much joy into my life (as have my older niece and nephew, and two baby nephews), and still does every time I see or even think about her. She's wonderful, as all children are. However, one particular day she taught me a very valuable lesson—and she was barely a year old at the time... It was a lesson I needed to learn about life, laughter, love, and opening your heart to the moment and the joys children bring into your life, regardless of whether they're your own or not.

I've always loved children. There's something about their carefree, innocent ways that makes me smile.

And it was on one particular day that the child was the teacher, and I the student.

Feeling beat up and worn by the stresses I sometimes let get the best of me, I made my way to my mother's house to take over babysitting my nine-month-old niece, Madeline. I arrived feeling like a wound up ball of string, unable to take in a deep, relaxing breath.

Shortly after I arrived, my mother left to go teach, and I was alone with Madeline. Remembering my mother said she was a bit fussy (she had four teeth coming in at once), I wondered what would keep her happy. The piano struck me as a good idea so I picked her up and carried her into the piano room.

Sitting on my lap, she composed her own 'masterpiece' as I watched in amazement. Babies have an uncanny ability to simply 'know' what to do. I didn't have to show her how to press the keys to create sound. She just knew.

After that, I decided to heat up a bottle for her. My mother said she may want one, so off to the kitchen we went.

In short order, the bottle was warmed enough and I carried her into the living room. Propping a pillow on the corner of the couch, I sat her down against it so she was nestled in safely. Covering her lap with a beautiful handmade baby blanket, I handed her the bottle, and she contentedly began to drink. But, not without a big, beautiful smile at me first. I felt my heart warm as I smiled back.

What do babies watch on television? I wondered. Clicking though the channels, I found *Barney* and saw her eyes light up. Okay, I thought. This must be it!

As the show went on, I watched Madeline watch television. I loved how she responded to the different songs and sights. There were so many expressions on her wee face.

I got so caught up in watching her that I didn't realize I'd grown relaxed and was breathing easier. But, somewhere between *I Love You, You Love Me* and the next song, I found that my shoulders weren't as tight, my head didn't ache, and I felt so much better than I had when I'd arrived.

As we sat on the couch, side by side, Madeline finished her bottle. I took it from her and placed it on the coffee table. We continued to watch television, just Madeline and I. I felt her gently snuggle up to my side. I smiled as I looked down at her—her big, blue eyes still mesmerized by the screen. It was a blessed feeling to know that this wonderful child, my niece, just wanted to lean against me. It truly warmed my heart.

When the show was over, she looked at me and smiled. I smiled back and made those 'baby sounds' you make when playing with a child. She let out the biggest 'belly laugh' that I'd ever heard a baby make! That alone made me laugh—and it was a real laugh. The more she laughed, the more I did, and it didn't take long before she and I were simply laughing away!

My focus was completely on laughing, smiling, playing, and just enjoying the moment. Oh did we have fun!

My mother arrived to find us both on the couch, laughing and relaxing. After changing Madeline's diaper and getting her settled again, it was time for me to go home.

I kissed them both goodbye, headed for my car, and began the short drive to my house.

It was during that drive that my eyes began to water. I felt, for the first time in my life, *what* God meant when He said that we should see through the eyes of a child. It was like a lightbulb went off in my head, and I *finally understood* the power of that statement.

Through Madeline, I saw through the eyes of a child. Those eyes, I surmised, see things like this: Love unconditionally. Trust. Don't judge. Celebrate life! Laugh! Look at all of God's creations around you in wonder. Smile at someone—just because you want to! Don't worry about things that might happen—enjoy the *now!*

The eyes of a child don't have to be 'taught' to see things this way. They just do.

In that short afternoon together, Madeline taught me what took 36 years to forget.

Thoughts on Celebrating the Now—(It's all you've got!)

It's very difficult to see all the blessings in your life when your stuck in the middle of a very dark, sad time. After my miscarriage, I nearly lost the ability to see the joy in everyday life or special events. I walked around in a state of sadness, longing, pain, regret—you name it. All these emotions, although very real, proved to be major obstacles in my being able to celebrate a joyful moment. It took a long time for me to learn that it was okay to laugh, smile, feel something beautiful when it happened. My whole way of thinking had to change. I had to allow myself to feel the good just as much as I was allowing myself to drown in the bad in order to provide some much needed balance in my life. The scales were tipped far too much in the wrong direction. I think this is normal for anyone after any loss, but if it goes on for too long, it's easy to fall deeper and deeper into a perpetual state of negativity and sadness, perhaps even depression. I know because I let it happen to me. So, I share this story to demonstrate how important it is to experience each second as it happens, without dwelling on the past or worrying about the future. Easier said than done, but very important nonetheless.

One thing I've discovered about myself as I stand at the late-thirties point of my life, is that I'm becoming more aware of celebrating the *now.* When I do, my soul feels nurtured. When I don't, I feel a hollowness deep within.

I wasn't very aware of the 'now' in my twenties. As I look back, I lived day to day, thinking things would go a certain way, and although there were times I relished a moment, I, more often than not, blew through them.

Time has taught me that there are many 'nows' that aren't so wonderful. They mean something, but it can be painful (emotionally) or simply not what you'd like the 'now' to be.

I have a problem with letting the issues of yesterday, or even five minutes ago, spoil a potentially joyous 'now.' However, I'm learning that by not allowing yourself to feel joy over something because you're upset at or by something else, you're depriving your soul of nourishment. Example: I have an argument with my partner and I can't let go of the feelings it caused. The argument may be over, but I carry resent or get hung up on 'whatever' being unresolved. Then, something great happens. I get some good news in the mail or over the phone. If I don't let go of what happened prior to that and the feelings associated with it, how can I possibly enjoy the newly revised 'now'? It's tough. I can't let things remain unresolved, but I can't let them ruin a wonderful thing that is worthy of celebration!

It's a trap I've allowed myself to fall into so many times, and one that my soul is screaming at me to end. Letting go doesn't mean that I'm rolling over or living in denial. It means that I know there are things in my life which need addressing, I have to address them, but I can't let them destroy the feelings I get when something joyous happens.
As I continue on my path to the soul, I hope to nurture it more by letting the good in and letting the bad go.

Thoughts on Letting it Go—Don't Let Your Balloon *Pop!*

Holding everything in serves no other purpose than to hurt you. There are times you need to let it out, whether you talk to a good friend, a therapist, write, talk to God—whatever you're comfortable with. After a miscarriage, there's a wealth of confusing thoughts playing through your mind, draining you of energy, making you wonder where you went. Please don't let them eat you up inside. Talk it out, let it out, set them free so you can take more steps forward on your journey to emotional, physical, and spiritual healing after miscarriage. Some days you're not fine, and even if you didn't suffer a miscarriage, there'd be days like that. If you get to a point where all you can think about is your miscarriage and you can't let go of any of the feelings that are causing anxiety, depression, bursts of crying, withdrawal, and more, please seek some professional help. It doesn't mean you're taking a step backwards.

It means you've got the courage to take a step forward—reclaiming your life.

I've come to the conclusion that it's okay to be 'not fine.'

When people ask me how I'm doing lately, I don't rattle off a list of complaints and observations, sad feelings and grievances—as a matter of fact, I just might say, "I'm okay." However, I admit that within myself things are *not* fine and try to work through the feelings that creates.

I don't need to share with others all of the time. It's good to vent to a friend and I don't discount that. But, I've learned that I'd better vent with myself and acknowledge my feelings or I, like a balloon with too much air, will *pop*.

Embrace the good and the not so good in your life. Don't run from it or try to bury it.

By doing this, by saying to myself that I am *not* fine right now, I can work through my feelings more easily.

How do I do it? It's taken me while to figure it out and I don't have all the answers. But, 'self-allowance' is very important.

I'm not advocating *dwelling* on your problems. I'm suggesting that you allow yourself to *feel*. The world isn't always sunshine and smiles, and if you try to force yourself into that very high, unrealistic expectation, you'll eventually *pop!*

I've done it, so I know.

You've got to let some air out of your balloon.

Give the air to God.

So, I acknowledge and embrace these parts of myself right now. I allow myself to feel hurt and cry. I turn to God for help and guidance, and I ask for more strength.

Here are some examples:

(I wrote this before my fiance's father passed away.)

My heart is ripped apart because my fiance's Dad was diagnosed with cancer. I *hate* being in the hospital seeing him suffer. I *detest* the fear that I feel and see and smell. I want to fall apart when I see the pain in my fiance's eyes. I am *not* okay with this. It hurts, and it hurts a lot. I cannot always be the pillar of strength I have expected myself to be. I lose it sometimes, and I am finally saying to myself that it's okay to do that. I ask God to help me. I need His strength so that I can be strong.

If I don't, my balloon will *pop*.

I can't always 'be there' without replenishing my resources. I don't have unlimited strength. I need time alone to embrace myself and my needs. I have to recharge my batteries so that I *can* be there for others.

119

I cannot do it alone. I am not meant to be the Energizer Bunny because I am human.

It *does* get to me when I see a patient in a hospital being mistreated, and I *do care*, and I *will* do something about it no matter what anyone else says. Example: I saw a man being wheeled by one nurse, while the other tagged behind with his IV. The nurse with the IV stopped, and the other kept going. Obviously this resulted in a lot of discomfort for the patient as the lines got tangled around his neck. He had to say, "Hey, what are you doing?" The nurses laughed. I had to let air out of my balloon. It was wrong. I couldn't keep still and silently watch this. The man's pillow fell to the floor, and the nurses were too busy laughing to realize the patient was struggling to get comfortable. Finally, one of them saw the pillow and plunked it *beside* his head, not under it. They didn't *care,* and that bothered me. My balloon was filling fast. How did I let some air out? I took action. I did what I knew was right in my gut. I walked up behind the man and said, while grabbing his pillow, "Do you need help with this?"

"Yes," he replied.

Big deal. I put the pillow under his head, and he was comfortable. He doesn't know whether I was a nurse or a stranger. It doesn't matter. He felt better and so did I. I helped, *but* why didn't the nurses?

I won't settle for that anymore. I can't save the world, but I can do my part.

That's letting air out of my balloon, too.

I've learned that when life gets too heavy, it doesn't mean you're *weak* if you admit it. It took a long time for me to get there. Tears don't equate to weakness. They are God's way of allowing you to cleanse your soul. I always had this crazy idea that if you can't handle things, you're weak. That's bologna.

That's what God is for.

So, let air out of your balloon. Cry if you have to. Help if you feel it's needed but are afraid of doing it. Voice a complaint if you have one. Allow yourself to 'be.' Let yourself know that you need to recharge once in a while and accept the fact that it's okay to let the injustices you see bother you. More importantly, do something about them if you can. Accept that you get tired and need to nurture yourself, too. If you're running around caring for others, know that it's draining and that there's only so much you can take before your balloon starts to fill too much. Don't punish yourself for needing rest. *Rest.* Let go of the guilt. Guilt fills balloons very quickly.

If a balloon has the right amount of air in it, it's beautiful, light, floating, colorful, and vibrant. Just like you.

Thoughts on Finding Joy in Holidays—
When Everything 'Feels' Wrong

I'll never forget that first Christmas after my miscarriage. My baby was supposed to have been born in November, and I was so excited about spending our very first holiday together as a family. As Christmas approached and there was no baby, I grew more and more depressed. The mere act of putting up a tree and decorating held little appeal. Everything about the holidays only served to magnify my pain, my loss, my grief. It was only after reconnecting to the significance and true meaning of Christmas that I was able to experience the joy of it. That doesn't mean I didn't have moments when I cried or sunk deeper into my darkened world. Of course it happened. But, I found the joy in Christmas when I allowed the message of love, hope, and healing back into my somewhat closed heart. I happen to celebrate Christmas, but, this applies to any holiday you celebrate—whatever faith you practice. Simply overlap the message I've shared into your own life and beliefs: Find the reason for the holiday and focus on it. *It's my greatest hope that you won't merely get through the holidays. I pray that you'll feel moments of healing joy and light.*

As you are surrounded by the sights and sounds of the holidays, you may show a bittersweet smile while gazing at lovely lights or hearing a children's choir. Perhaps you feel guilty for feeling happy when inside you've been reflecting on all the wishes and dreams you had for your baby and how much you would have loved to have spent the holidays with your special little one.

It may feel like the holiday spirit has been knocked out of your sails and you're drifting aimlessly upon a sea of tears.

Yes, you've experienced a terrible loss. Sometimes the feelings seems incomprehensible and insurmountable. You're left wondering how to get through any celebration with joy in your heart. Where is the room for joy when your heart is filled to the brim with sorrow?

So many times my eyes misted when I thought of the baby I wouldn't be holding when Christmas came. It seemed nothing could take away my pain, turn back the clocks, make life the way I wanted it to be. Where was my baby? Why did this happen? How can I even celebrate when I'm feeling so sad? I asked myself these questions over and over again until they became part of who I was.

My attempts of feeling joy during a season that was supposed to be joyous were futile, until something changed in my *thinking*.

As I battled with guilt and sorrow, I wondered if I should even bother decorating for Christmas the year I miscarried. I was caught, literally, in a web of grief and self pity. It was very destructive.

I asked myself, "What right do I have to be happy?"

One day, quite out of the blue, I came to the conclusion that it was okay, even necessary to experience the joy and hope of the holidays that year. If I could take my focus away from *my* problems and point it towards what Christmas (in my case), really was—I knew I'd find comfort, solace, peace, and joy. To me, Christmas is God and God is eternal love, hope, life, joy, and peace. Isn't that what I needed more than ever?

By focusing on God—my burdens became lighter and I saw the message of great hope and comfort. No, my pain wasn't gone. No, I couldn't bring back the baby I never held. I couldn't reverse time. But, there is no load too heavy that God won't carry for me, for you, if that's what you believe. Through God and His message, I took comfort in many things during the holiday season. First, the baby I lost was indeed living with our loving Father in an alive, eternal, and beautiful world. Though not with me physically, my baby was very much alive and happy. The heartache was there, my baby missed dearly, but knowing in my heart he lived on put the holiday wind back in my sails. Second, no matter how heavy my load was, God was always there to help me with it. His gift of hope, comfort, help, healing and life sustained me, brought me through and into the light celebration. I was carried through my darkest hours. I was never alone. There was someone right beside me who would see me through anything the world decided to dish out. Third, the light of God shines within each and every one of us. The beauty of lights upon a tree or shining from a Menorah symbolize His omnipresent light. As I struggled with whether or not I should put decorations up—I remembered what they symbolized. They are symbols of the light of God and cannot ever be snuffed out. By displaying lights and decorations, I was not only showing hope to myself for a brighter tomorrow, but also gave hope to others who may have needed to be reminded of it very, very much.

It is my hope that you can, even with your very real pain, not just 'get through' your holiday season, but celebrate it. Now more than ever you need reconnect to what Christmas, or whatever holiday you celebrate, truly means. In doing that, you will find joy, even if it's amidst tears.

May the light of God shine in all of your hearts, giving you comfort, peace and joy.

"Peace on Earth. Good will toward men."

Thoughts on Fear and Faith: Fear is Faith Inverted

During periods of great loss, it's only natural to question your faith. I did. So many of us wonder how God could 'let this happen'—be it your miscarriage or any other personal or global tragedy. If your faith is being tested right now, as mine was, you may want to read on. People tend to blame God when things go wrong. I know I did—and it was tough for me to admit. I knew better; yet, something inside of me was holding onto the thought that God could have prevented my miscarriage. It was only after a great deal of time passed that I realized there's a reason for everything, even things that hurt deeply. I don't blame God for my miscarriage. I know there were reasons, unknown to me, for it. While I was in my blaming mode, I was full of fear. When I learned to trust in God, my fear was transformed into faith. That doesn't mean the pain went away. It means by having faith instead of fear, the pain of my miscarriage was lessened because I knew my baby was in heaven, and I needed to lean on Him to get through the very tough times and beyond. My fear also led to an inability to relax (and still does when I let it take over faith's place). Fear is natural; it's what you do with it that will determine how well you fare during any time of crisis in your life. Not only times of crisis, but everyday living, too. I wish you more faith than fear.

The first thing to come to mind at this moment is this saying: Fear is faith inverted. I think there's a lot of truth to that. I have a lot of faith, and it's carried me through some of the rockiest times of my life. But, I'm human and I feel, cut, bleed, and cry like the rest of us. And no matter how much faith I have, there are those moments when I simply "lose it" and am scared out of my mind. It feels like all my faith is gone. Thank God that after these moments, I sense the gentle hand of God calming me down, and I know that everything is going to work out...somehow.

But, why can't I just have faith all the time and avoid those moments where I can't give my life to God completely? Why do I sometimes get paralyzed with fear? I don't know. I guess it's because I just haven't learned to do it yet. I wonder if anyone ever can. Are there people out there who are so confident and full of faith that they never become fearful? I'm not one of them.

The other day we found out that a family member has cancer. At least that's the first call the doctor who did the examination made. As far as I am concerned, the jury is still out until the biopsy results come in. I prayed and prayed and am still praying. I am visualizing the body healing itself through the light of God, and I am boldly asking for a miracle. Why not? I have the right to, just like anyone else. The thing about miracles is this: You have to believe in them for them to happen. I do, and I am not afraid to ask for one because I've gotten over the 'I don't deserve to ask for one' stage of my life. God wants me to ask, He wants to give, and He wants me to believe that He can and will help. So, I asked for one.

However, fear rears its ugly head once again, and I find myself alone and crying. I am saying, "God, please help me to be strong. Please—help—me."

Another family member, my Dad, is scheduled for an echocardiogram. Wait a minute! My Dad? An echocardiogram? No, this can't be. He's my father! No, he can't have a heart problem. No way. He's the guy who plays the piano like there's no tomorrow and is my musical hero. He's the guy I gigged with for the first time at sixteen. He's active. People love him.

God, what's happening? I am afraid again. Where'd my faith go? Is it still there? If it is, why am I so full of fear? It's too much at once, God. I need your help. Please help turn my fear into faith. Please help me to take comfort in You. God, please help me walk the walk and not just talk the talk.

And then I realize that it's okay to be afraid. It's normal. If I weren't ever scared, I don't think I'd be human. And through that fear comes faith. It's a metamorphosis of sorts. *If not for the fear, I wouldn't turn to God for help. That act of turning is faith.*

Thoughts On Self-Forgiveness—I Wasn't There

I share this story with you for one reason: We can't control the uncontrollable, and to blame ourselves for our miscarriage is extremely self-destructive. The following example of self-blame and learning to let go of something that wasn't my fault, my grandmother's death, is shared with the genuine hope that if you're beating yourself up for miscarrying, you'll stop. Please—for your own good.

In March of 1986, I was struggling through my sophomore year of college, was twenty years old, had just become engaged, and was living the life of busy person wrapped up in their own world. I remember March seventeenth very well, but not because it was St. Patty's Day. At the time, my older sister lived near campus, and I would often go to her house in between classes. My niece and nephew were babies, and it was a nice break from the day. My father called. I remember it was warm out because we were sitting outside. Yes, it was warm for March in New England.

I remember my father saying, "Are you sitting down?" When you hear that, you know it isn't good.

"No, but I will. What's up, Dad?"

"Your Grammy died."

"What? When?"

This is the part of the story that I've always had difficulty with. This is the part of my story where self-forgiveness became a huge issue with me. For this is the part of my story where I'd discovered that my Grammy, my sweet ex-Broadway star Grammy, had been dead for three days before *anyone* knew.

"One of her friends called the police after not seeing her for a few days."

I was numb. Three days? I just went on living my life as if everything was fine while my grandmother lay dead on the floor of her apartment for three days. Phone contact was all we had. She lived in Connecticut, and I still lived at home with my parents. Whenever she called, I'd talk to her. She wanted to know everything that was going on. I told her about my Theatre classes and my voice and diction class. I told her I was trying to get rid of my Massachusetts accent, and she said, "Oh, don't do that." I told her I was engaged and she was happy. She sounded great. I asked her how everything was in her new apartment that I hadn't seen.

"Everything's fine."

Everything *wasn't* fine.

She was always a proud woman. After losing her husband when my mother was just seven months old, she worked and sent my mother to the New England Conservatory of Music. She was strong, capable, and talented. She'd also never ask for help. Ever.

I remember our yearly trips to her house near the ocean every summer. A picture of perfection. Everything in her home was perfect. Perfectly neat, clean, organized. Beds always made; no dust anywhere. The furniture she'd had for years was still in the same perfect shape as it was when my mother was a child. She was the picture of perfection. Always well dressed, well groomed with beautiful hair as white and shiny as newly fallen snow. Her nails were always painted a soft, luminescent color. She lived alone after my mother went off to college. She didn't have her parents around anymore. She did everything herself, including riding her bike to the local convenience store to get what she needed. That's how she was. Independent.

She sold her lovely white Dutch Colonial with the red trim that her father built and moved into a small, brick-faced apartment building. It was one of those places where the elderly lived. I never saw it, well, until she was gone.

The trip to Connecticut after she died was horrible. I didn't know what to expect or how to feel. I was consumed with guilt but that wouldn't compare to the guilt I would feel after seeing her apartment.

My parents arrived a day before my sister and I. We met them at the hotel, and they told us to be prepared. "For what?"

I knew what they meant when we got there. The moment we walked in the stink was so bad I felt I was going to be ill. That was after my parents had the windows open overnight. After it had aired out. The sink had dishes in it that were there for God knows how long. The apartment she'd lived in for two years was strewn with boxes that still remained unpacked. All of her things were packed away except for the bare necessities. This was the same woman who *had* to have everything perfect and who *never* asked for help.

Oh God, Grammy, why didn't you say anything? I would have been there. Mom would have been there. We all would have been there to help you settle in. I know we were busy, but why didn't you ask? Why didn't I offer?

There it is. Why didn't I offer? Why didn't I know? Why didn't I call more often and pick up that something wasn't right? Why didn't I drive down to Connecticut on breaks and see her? Why was I so absorbed in my life that I didn't realize she was suffering in silence? How could I have let my grandmother live that way? How?

She seemed to know exactly what she was doing. Although most of her things were packed away, she left out, as if on purpose, some beautiful jewelry for my mother to find. She left some very important paperwork out for my mother to find. Such obvious places amongst all the clutter. So clearly defined. So easy to see, while everything else looked like a scrambled puzzle of old boxes and furniture.

Why didn't the people who delivered her groceries ever *call* and tell my mother how she was living? Couldn't they see she wasn't using most of the things they brought that she was paying for? Or did they just care about getting their money? I don't know. I can't look to them. I can't place any responsibility on them even though it would help to relieve my own feelings of it. No, they weren't family.

So, all these years have passed. Fourteen, going on fifteen now. Have I forgiven myself? I've reflected a lot. The nightmares went away. I've felt connected to Grammy spiritually in a very strong way. I feel her presence. I talk to her and have researched her life. I still love her. I have learned that I cannot blame myself for being twenty and living like someone who was twenty. I know if the same circumstances existed today, I would be there, I would call, I would make sure everything was okay. But that can't happen.

Sometimes it's easier to forgive others than it is to forgive ourselves. Over time, I think I've forgiven myself. I've heard Grammy say to me, "It wasn't your fault." I've struggled with regret, but know it's a dangerous thing to carry around. I've learned that blaming myself for Grammy's death would be like blaming myself for my miscarriage. There was nothing I could do about it, and it was completely out of my hands.

When Nana (my Dad's mother) took a turn for the worse, *I was there.* All the time, trying to feed her, trying to instill in her the will to live that she'd lost. I know that it's in me to be there. It was in me back in 1986, too. I just didn't know I was needed.

You can't spend your whole life kicking yourself for something you wish you'd done differently. I know that much. That comes with time. I can't change the fact that I was twenty and had a different take on life. I was in acceleration mode and just took for granted that everyone in my family was fine. Yes, I forgive myself. It wasn't easy to do; and I've grown a lot in the process.

Note: We are often much harder on ourselves than God is. I believe that over time He helped me to treat myself more gently—as He always does.

Thoughts on Finding Your Key to Happiness: Once Upon a Time

Don't forget who you are. You are a beautiful creation, your dreams are real, and although easy to set them aside and settle for less, it's a sad thing to do. Often, you forget how to be happy or where to find happiness. Remember, it lies within yourself. For years I let my happiness remain on the back burner. It doesn't matter why; what matters is what it did to me. I became someone I hardly recognized anymore. My dreams lie dormant within me, and the longer I ignored them, the more uneasy I became. Life began to feel like an uncomfortable shoe—because I was ignoring my essence. We all grow up and have responsibilities. That doesn't mean you can't dream and reach for that dream. Perhaps it'll be modified, but it's yours and it's you.

Once upon a time a baby girl was born. She knew her destiny, for it was embedded within her heart and mind. As she grew older and experienced life, her destiny became foggy. The girl became wrapped up in the world and searched for happiness there among friends and material things.

As a teenager, she experienced all of the trials and tribulations that went along with youth. She distanced herself from her parents, tested the waters of independence, and she distanced herself from her soul, believing that she would find what her heart yearned for outside of herself.

As a young woman in college, she studied what she wanted to and applied little effort to that which didn't interest her. Somewhere within the recesses of her mind she knew she could do better, but she couldn't find where the nagging feeling was coming from. So, she squeaked by, disappointed in herself for not doing better.

She married, and the marriage failed. She did not find the happiness she so longed for within her partner; nor did he find it within her. They were both lost—yet their road was so close.

Time passed and the young woman, now in her thirties, began to sense that something was buried deep with herself. A key of sorts, which she had to find. It brought back feelings of her youth but she didn't know why. It seemed to her that her world was so clear back then. Wanting clarity, she began her quest, not knowing what she was looking for or where she was going.

As if being guided by an external force, she was led to various clues upon her journey. Many of those clues came in the form of books. Over time, she found herself gravitating to topics such as spiritualism, philosophy, healing, and senses beyond what we have deemed our only five. Much reading took place over the next several years. Engulfed on a journey to her soul, she kept delving into whatever she could find that made sense to her, coming closer and closer to the key that lay dormant within her heart. After many hours, days, weeks, months and years, she learned something that would change her life forever.

Instead of asking "why" when a painful situation arose in her life, she began asking herself, "What can I learn from this? What am I supposed to know?" She learned to still herself and tune out the external. Her focus became on the internal, on her heart and soul.

It was there that she discovered, after many painful years and lessons, that the key to happiness does not lie within the 'world' outside of ourselves or within another. She learned that the key to her happiness was within her own heart, as was her destiny. She needed to still herself long enough to listen to what the universe had been trying to tell her all along. Follow what you believe is right for you, what you know is right for you. Listen to your heart, and heed your soul's messages.

Ever thankful for the lesson she'd learned, she continued on her journey, knowing that she had just begun to realize what it would take to make herself truly 'happy.' Along her road, she shared with others who wanted to know, who wanted to hear. It made her heart sing when they understood, and her heart wept when they did not. However, she realized that although we are all connected, we do not learn the same things at the same time. We all have our own road to travel. We all have our own key to find. Our own key to happiness.

Thoughts on Counting Your Blessings—Out of the Box

This is a fictional story, but I share it because sometimes I've forgotten to count how many blessings are in my life, especially when going through a very difficult, painful time. By focusing on the needs of others in more dire circumstances, we often come to realize that although our pain is very real, there are so many others who literally have nothing but the shirts on their backs. With this realization comes the ability to see past the fog of our own personal grief and feel grateful for things even as basic as a roof over our heads, food, people who love us. In the wake of Hurricane Katrina (and all other disasters in 2005, worldwide), thoughts of appreciation become more clear. I know it's all relative, and we all have our own pains. But, we all have our own happiness, too, and when we lose the ability to see or feel what makes us happy, it's time to step out of ourselves and look at the world around us. We'll see many things, two of them being: There are others far worse off than you. And, there's so much beauty in your life and in the world around you to experience and appreciate.

Maddy huddled in her latest treasure to keep warm. The softness of the fur, although matted and worn in some spots, was to her the epitome of luxury. As her hands clung tightly to it, she realized that this was no ordinary find and would be desirable to many. It must stay with her at all times or she would come 'home' one day to find it missing.

Curling up into a small ball, in fetal position, Maddy could see hundreds of feet walking by. The bodies to which they belonged didn't know she was there—watching and freezing. It was a typical busy Boston evening. Folks scurried from the train station hurrying to the theater district. All Maddy saw was their feet and wondered what it would be like to have nice shoes and a place to go. Even more so, she tried to remember what it felt like to have a warm place to go afterwards. A place called home. How long she'd been living in this box was unknown. If forever could be measured, surely this was the gauge.

A cold wind found its way into her abode, causing her to shiver. She thanked God for her newly found treasure. Yes, it had been a good day of hunting. She'd managed to find the coat, a mismatched pair of wool socks, and, although men's, a pair of winter boots. They were big and heavy on her small feet, but kept them warm.

She curled up into an even smaller ball and tried to sleep. The pangs of hunger kept her awake as she watched the world walk by. She'd been late to the shelter, and there wasn't any food left, save a piece of bread. At least she got that. One of her street friends was kind enough to share a piece of cheese with her, as well. Maddy knew she'd return the favor. That's how it worked here. Her eyes grew heavy as the lull of soles on pavement echoed in her ears. Finally, sleep came and took her away from her box into a different world. A world with clean, crisp white curtains and a large yard. A world with children playing on a swingset and the smell of a wonderful roast in the oven. A world of clean laundry neatly folded in baskets waiting to be put away. A world with a husband who came home and they all sat to dinner, laughing, and eating. A world that was shattered after the accident.

They were gone in the blink of an eye. He kissed her goodbye that morning, taking the children to school on his way to work, and she never saw them again. He never saw the truck skidding on the ice. Her life was buried beneath the earth.

Then she 'lost it.' After that, she lost her job and her home. With no job came no insurance and no medication. Her family was gone, and those she thought were friends weren't. She found herself on the street in a fraction of a second. She didn't care at first—about anything. Survival meant nothing because she had nothing to survive for.

Days turned into weeks and weeks into months, and now it had been two years of living in a box.

She awoke in the morning, her dream still fresh in her mind and a tear gently rolled down her dirty face. *The only difference,* she thought, as she looked at the polished shoes walking by her box, *between them and me is that they don't know what they have—and they haven't lost it.*

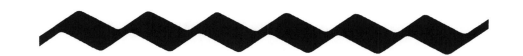

Parting Thoughts

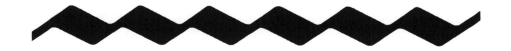

Parting Thoughts—But Not Parting Ways

I know you're living in a world right now that sometimes doesn't seem real. It's too scary, lonely, and sad to be your life. You hardly recognize it anymore. I know that feeling. It's like a nightmare no one can wake you from, because you're already awake.

I know what it's like to be sitting on the couch, driving in my car, walking through the supermarket—and feel a sudden onslaught of tears. I've lived those days when you don't know if you've got the strength to hold them back.

I know what it's like to sit on the couch with your hands resting on your now empty womb, crying so hard over what could have been that your body hurts afterwards. My mind flashed to images of what my baby would have looked like, what his room would have been like, how he would have felt in my arms. I remained stuck in that painful spot for a very long time, and I know what it feels like to think you'll never escape from it—to wonder where the life jacket is and who's going to throw it.

I know what it's like to feel ashamed for feeling jealous of women who had healthy, beautiful babies—after I just lost mine. I felt the guilt—knew it was wrong, but couldn't stop myself from feeling it.

I know what it's like to feel angry at my spouse for not understanding me more. I know what it's like to be snappy and cold, even when your heart tells you it's not how you want to be—not what you meant to say. You want to scream out, "I'm in pain, that's why I'm acting this way!" But you don't, and the cycle continues. Sometimes the distance between you becomes overwhelming, and it's exactly the opposite of what your heart craves. Yet, you don't know how to ask to be close—what to say, how to feel.

I know what it's like to retrace every one of your footsteps to see what you did wrong to cause your miscarriage. I dwelled on the glasses of wine I had before I knew I was pregnant and on the cigarettes I smoked before I knew I was pregnant. I went through my life with a fine tooth comb so I could find a reason, any reason, for my miscarriage. I never found any, but tortured myself just the same.

I know what it's like to go to a baby shower and feel like running from the room because I couldn't take the pain of being around people who were so joyful and had every right to be. I know about feeling like a third wheel when your friends or acquaintances all have healthy babies or pregnancies and you're left living through the nightmare of not having your own baby to love.

I know what it's like to turn to God and instead of praying, blaming Him for your miscarriage. I did it—I asked why, and when I thought I didn't get an answer, I felt even more alone. I couldn't see, couldn't feel anything but my own pain, and when God didn't make it all go away, I got angry and sad. I felt guilty for it feeling that way and beat myself up for that, too. I drove myself into an even deeper hole.

I know what it's like to be afraid to be intimate again, for fear of another pregnancy—or loss of one. I felt the conflicting emotions of wanting a baby so badly, yet after having suffered such a loss, being too paralyzed by the fear of it happening again. *What if it happened again? I couldn't take it.* Those thoughts have run through my mind.

I know what it's like to pull out the one baby outfit you allowed yourself to buy from its secret hiding space and clutch it tightly to your chest, tears streaming down your face as you think of the baby who will never fill it. I also know what it's like to let go of that outfit, giving it to a friend who just found out she's pregnant—telling yourself over and over that you're doing the right thing. She will use it. She'll have a healthy baby. At the same time, feelings of jealousy, sadness, and resentment combined with happiness for your friend. It was confusing and tiring, lonely and scary.

I know how much I allowed my self esteem to get beat up after I miscarried. I put on some weight, couldn't stand myself for it (even though I was four and a half months pregnant when I miscarried), and felt simply terrible about myself. I couldn't find the motivation to exercise, to eat right, to make myself feel better because I was too busy grieving, when no one else was grieving with me—or at least I didn't think they were.

I know how frightening it is when your heart suddenly races and it scares you out of your mind. I felt like I was going to have a heart attack, choke, or die. I know how scary feelings of anxiety can be. When you don't know what anxiety is, it's even more terrifying. I felt like I was going crazy and would never be the 'old' me again. I lost the old me.

I know what it's like to love the baby you never got to hold.

But there's something else I know.

I know that over time you will heal, smile again, feel like your old self, and be able to live your life. I know that you will be able to hold a friend's baby or celebrate the pregnancy of someone without feeling resentful. I know you'll be able to shop for baby clothes again and smile because they're so cute. I know you'll be able to stop blaming yourself, God, or anyone else for your miscarriage. I know you'll begin to flourish and experience new and beautiful things in your life. I know there'll come a time when you won't feel like crying every ten seconds. I know you'll be able to accompany someone to an ultrasound and actually get through it in one piece. I know time will become your friend, not your enemy. I know you'll be able to feel the joy and wonder when a baby looks into your eyes and smiles. I know the wall you've built around your heart will be torn down, one brick at a time.

I know this, because I am there. I have my moments when I slip back into that dreadful time—the time when I miscarried, and I'll never forget it or my baby in heaven. But, when I think of the dark, isolated place I was in and compare that to where I am today, I see the impossible happened—I journeyed down a road of healing and recovery.

I also know, more than anything else, that after your journey you will be able to offer comfort to a woman who's miscarried. The world will become a place where miscarriage is not something that's simply brushed aside as a non-event, and you will have the strength and courage to offer your hand out to a sister in need during her darkest hours.

Together, we can make a difference. Together, we can provide hope and healing—instead of isolation and fear. We can show women everywhere that they are not alone in their suffering. With our arms outstretched we can say, "I have lived it, I am here for you." After crying our own tears, we can dry the tears of those crying now.

Our babies never got to see this earth, but we can take comfort that our angel babies are just that—angels. Although we can't see them, we can feel them in us, around us, and you will always be able to say, "I am that baby's mother." Because, you are.

Through adversity comes strength. I'd never wish this kind of adversity on you, but since you are living it, you can take it and turn it into something that will not only make you a stronger person, but will enable you to lend some strength to those who need it. Maybe not today or even this year—but, someday.

Gone are they days when the woman who miscarried is denied the chance to grieve, feel, hope, and heal. Through our sharing, we create awareness. Through awareness, comes the masses saying, "I feel that way, too. Yes, I need some help to get through this." And women will get the help they need.

Fifteen years ago I walked into a bookstore hoping, praying to find a book that told me I wasn't crazy for feeling how I did after I miscarried. A book that spoke to me and didn't tell me why I miscarried, but simply let me know that I'd be okay and offered me some help. I couldn't find a book like that, no matter where I turned. It is a new day, and my greatest wish for any woman who's suffered a miscarriage is that she'll walk into a bookstore seeking support from a book, and she'll pick up this one. Through my story—which is really *all of our stories*— the wonderful, heartfelt words of Dr. Linda Backman, Anna Pizzoferrato, and the other beautiful women who shared their hearts in this book, the woman who has miscarried will finally find what I longed for so long ago. *Hope.*

The Angel In You

You don't see her, but I do.
Each time your eyes twinkle
I see her in you.
Every time you wipe my tears
with your kind and gentle ways—
I see in you an Angel
sent to smooth the way.
I don't know what I did
to deserve such a friend.
I thank God for you, my dear one—
My Angel until the end.
I hope that when you look
to me for comfort and for Love—
you see in me an Angel
sent from up above.
It's the part of us that's giving,
the part that's so refined—
The part that's made of only Love—
The part that is Divine.
We are Angels to each other
whenever we lend a hand—
or dry a tear or soothe a wound—
it's all part of the plan.
Reach inside your heart
and you will surely find;
part of you that is an Angel—
so loving, warm and kind.

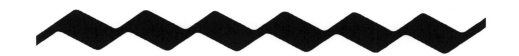

Resources

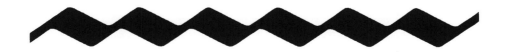

Miscarriage Resources on the Internet

The following websites offer wonderful support if you're suffering from a miscarriage and its fallout. I strongly advocate turning to these sites if you need someone to talk to who understands what you're living. The doors to the world have been literally kicked open by the Internet, allowing us access where we once had none. Please take advantage of these resources if you're able and peace to you on your way.

I've done my best to ensure these websites still exist; however, the Internet is constantly changing. If you find a site is no longer there, my apologies.

MiscarriageHelp.com is the companion website to this book. It is a place where you can post your feelings about miscarriage with others, have a safe place to vent, take comfort in sharing with those who know what you're living, read comforting articles, and/or post your own to help others.
http://www.MiscarriageHelp.com

Ravenheart Center
Dr. Linda Backmanis dedicated to psychospiritual healing in the areas of death/loss/grief.
http://www.ravenheartcenter.com

Reiki With Trust LLC, Distance Energy Healing
Anna Pizzoferrato is there for those times, events, or situations that could use some extra help.
http://www.ReikiWithTrust.com/

KotaPress offers support and outreach to families enduring the death of a child and to the caregivers who are with those families. Outreach happens through the free online *Loss Journal* at www.KotaPress.com, a print zine. "A Different Kind of Parenting: a zine for parents whose

children have died, our Mrs. Duck Project, and more."
http://www.kotapress.com

Angel Babies Forever Loved offers support to grieving parents of infants. Whether from miscarriage, stillbirth, neonatal loss, or SIDS, we all share in the loss of our babies.
http://www.angels4ever.com/

The Compassionate Friends mission is to assist families toward the positive resolution of grief following the death of a child of any age and to provide information to help others be supportive.
Toll-free: 877-969-0010
http://www.compassionatefriends.org
Email: nationaloffice@compassionatefriends.org

WomantoWoman—a women's community
http://women2women.com/

The MISS Foundation "is a nonprofit, volunteer-based organization committed to providing emergency support to families in crisis after the death of their baby or young child from any cause. We are here to help families cope with the resultant feelings of overwhelming grief and loss. We are committed to public awareness to decrease infant mortality; we support medical research committed to the same cause. Our vision is to perpetuate education and awareness on ethics and death issues; decreasing enigmas surrounding grief and increasing bereavement sensitivity, and crisis intervention protocol establishment through a psychosocial, multidisciplinary training program. No family should have to endure the trauma of a child's death alone: MISS is committed to the memory of the children who lived, who died, and who continue— even in death—to matter."
http://www.missfoundation.org/

OfSpirit.com Magazine is an online resource for education, entertainment, and empowerment in the holistic, spiritual, and self-improvement field. Find articles, interviews, links, and a weekly online magazine, on everything from Acupuncture to Zen.
http://www.ofspirit.com

The Center for Grieving Children A Place of Healing and Hope
http://www.grievingchildren.org/

Feelings of the Fathers
http://www.thelaboroflove.com/forum/loss/fathers.html

Sidelines National Support Network
http://www.sidelines.org/

Surviving Miscarriage
http://www.ferre.org/newbrow/infbroc/survive.html

Grief, Loss, Recovery
Articles, poems & personal stories about grief, loss, and recovery.
http://www.grieflossrecovery.com

Aumara Healing A Place for Healing and Inspiration
http://www.aumara.com/intro.html

"**Angels4ever** is a non-profit 501(c)3 corporation established to support grieving parents of infants. Whether from miscarriage, stillbirth, neonatal loss, or SIDS, we all share in the loss of our babies."
http://angels4ever.com/

Coping With a Miscarriage
Approved by the Baby Center Medical Advisory Board
http://www.babycenter.com/refcap/4006.html

The Bright Side can help if you or a loved one needs help but doesn't know where to go or what types of help are available, . On The Bright Side website you will find educational materials, articles by top experts, personal stories, and other resources to help you cope with depression, grief, suicide, or whatever mental or emotional difficulty you or your loved one may be experiencing. A little support can go a long way towards helping us cope and shedding light into our personal darkness.
http://www.the-bright-side.org

About the Author

Ellen DuBois lives in Massachusetts and is a multi-published author in the fiction, nonfiction, and poetry genres. She is slated to appear in several books in 2006-2008 and is currently working on her next projects.

Contacting the Author

Web: MiscarriageHelp.com
Web: EllenDuBois.com
Email: ellen@miscarriagehelp.com

Made in the USA
Middletown, DE
10 February 2015